CORPVS SPECVLORVM
ETRVSCORVM

CORPVS SPECVLORVM ETRVSCORVM

U.S.A. 1: MIDWESTERN COLLECTIONS

ANN ARBOR—KELSEY MUSEUM OF ARCHAEOLOGY, UNIVERSITY OF MICHIGAN
BLOOMINGTON—INDIANA UNIVERSITY ART MUSEUM
CHICAGO—ART INSTITUTE OF CHICAGO
CHICAGO—FIELD MUSEUM OF NATURAL HISTORY
CHICAGO—ORIENTAL INSTITUTE, UNIVERSITY OF CHICAGO
CINCINNATI—CINCINNATI ART MUSEUM
CLEVELAND—CLEVELAND MUSEUM OF ART
COLUMBIA—MUSEUM OF ART AND ARCHAEOLOGY, UNIVERSITY OF MISSOURI
CRAWFORDSVILLE—WABASH COLLEGE ANTIQUITIES COLLECTION
DAYTON—DAYTON ART INSTITUTE
DETROIT—DETROIT INSTITUTE OF ARTS
IOWA CITY—CLASSICAL MUSEUM, UNIVERSITY OF IOWA
KANSAS CITY—NELSON-ATKINS MUSEUM OF ART
LAWRENCE—WILCOX COLLECTION, UNIVERSITY OF KANSAS
MILWAUKEE—MILWAUKEE PUBLIC MUSEUM
MINNEAPOLIS—MINNEAPOLIS INSTITUTE OF ARTS
OBERLIN—ALLEN MEMORIAL ART MUSEUM, OBERLIN COLLEGE
OMAHA—JOSLYN ART MUSEUM
ROCKFORD—ROCKFORD COLLEGE ART COLLECTION
ST. LOUIS—ST. LOUIS ART MUSEUM
TOLEDO—TOLEDO MUSEUM OF ART

TEXT AND DRAWINGS BY

RICHARD DANIEL De PUMA

IOWA STATE UNIVERSITY PRESS—AMES—1987

Published with the assistance of the J. Paul Getty Trust

FIRST EDITION, 1987

Library of Congress Cataloging-in-Publication Data

Corpus speculorum etruscorum.

    Includes indexes.
    Contents: v. 1. Midwestern collections : text and drawings / by
Richard Daniel De Puma.
    1. Mirrors, Etruscan — Catalogs 2. Mirrors — United States —
Catalogs. 3. Italy — Antiquities — Catalogs.
I. De Puma, Richard Daniel, 1942–
DG223.7.M55D4   1987   739'.512'09375074013   86–
31135
ISBN 0–8138–0363–2 (v. 1)

TO MY MOTHER

CONTENTS

Addenda

ACKNOWLEDGEMENTS

Examining, photographing, and drawing Etruscan mirrors in twenty-one midwestern collections was an exhausting but educational experience. I envy my fellow Etruscologists who have the luxury of finding all their mirrors conveniently gathered together in one brightly lit museum storeroom. In several instances I have had to "excavate" the subjects treated in this fascicle from the dusty strata of museum magazines or retrieve them from the limbo of "Egyptian" storage. I have learned always to check Egyptian when looking for Etruscan. The results have been rewarding. Many pieces have found their rightful place, and I profited much from the exploration of areas normally ignored.

My numerous requests to the various staff members of these collections have usually been handled efficiently and promptly. I wish to record, with gratitude, the names of those who have assisted me: Elaine K. Gazda, John G. Pedley, and Pamela Reister (Ann Arbor); Adriana Calinescu, Danae Thimme, and Wolf Rudolph (Bloomington); John Carswell, Anita Ghaemi, Barbara Hall, and Robin Chamberlin (Chicago, Oriental Institute); Glen Cole, Lillian Novak, Phyllis Rabineau, and James VanStone (Chicago, Field Museum); Louise Berge, Mary Gruel, and R. Bret Ruiz (Chicago, Art Institute); Ingeborg Schweiger and Daniel Walker (Cincinnati); Arielle Kozloff, Jenifer Neils, Frederick Hollendonner, and Bruce Christman (Cleveland); Jane Biers and Saul Weinberg (Columbia); John Fischer (Crawfordsville); Kent Sobotek, Dominique Vasseur, and Susan Walsh (Dayton); William Peck, Gary Carriveau, and Timothy Motz (Detroit); Roger Hornsby (Iowa City); Ross Taggart, Forrest Bailey, and Ann Erbacher (Kansas City); Elizabeth Banks (Lawrence); Rudolph Dornemann, Arthur J. Frank, and John Lundstrom (Milwaukee); Michael Conforti and Catherine Asher (Minneapolis); Christine Dyer, Fred Albertson, Nancy Heller, and Mary Sturgeon (Oberlin); Berneal Anderson, Bernard Barryte, and Henry Flood Robert (Omaha); Raymond DenAdel, Philip Dedrick, and Louise Giliberti (Rockford); Sidney Goldstein, Diane Burke, and Betty Grossman (St. Louis); and Kurt Luckner (Toledo).

I consulted, quizzed, or annoyed a number of other students of Etruscan matters and thank them for their assistance, patience, and encouragement: Larissa Bonfante (New York), Nancy de Grummond (Tallahassee), Paul Denis (Toronto), Adriana Emiliozzi (Florence), Edilberto Formigli (Rome), Eleanor Guralnick (Chicago), Gerald Heres (Berlin), Ursula Höckmann (Mainz), Ines Jucker (Bern), Roger Lambrechts (Brussels), Neda Leipen (Toronto), Ursula Liepmann (Hannover), Glenys Lloyd-Morgan (Chester), Bettina von Freytag gen. Löringhoff (Tübingen), Torben Melander (Copenhagen), David Mitten

(Cambridge), Kyle M. Phillips, Jr. (Florence), Denise Rebuffat-Emmanuel (Paris), Emeline H. Richardson (Durham), Helle Salskov Roberts (Copenhagen), W. Rosenbaum (Ascona), Jocelyn Penny Small (New Brunswick), Judith Swaddling (London), Holger Termer (Hamburg), Jean M. Turfa (Philadelphia), Ellen Williams (Washington), and Ingela Wiman (Lund).

For their excellent technical assistance in analyzing the bronze samples for several mirrors, I am especially grateful to John Edie (University of Iowa Electron Microprobe Analysis Facility, Iowa City) and Lee Friell and Shamsher Brar (University of Iowa Hygienic Laboratory, Des Moines). Funds for this work were kindly provided by the Graduate College of the University of Iowa.

Finally, I am pleased to acknowledge the generous assistance, support, and encouragement of my friends and colleagues: Larissa Bonfante (New York University), Kyle M. Phillips, Jr. (Florence), Wallace J. Tomasini (University of Iowa), and Richard L. Sawyer (American College Testing, Iowa City). They helped to make this task much easier.

ABBREVIATIONS

Bibliographical Abbreviations

AEArq	*Archivo Español de Arqueologia*
AJA	*American Journal of Archaeology*
AnnInst	*Annali dell'Istituto di Corrispondenza Archeologica*
AntK	*Antike Kunst*
ArchCl	*Archeologia Classica*
ArchN	*Archeological News*
BClevMus	*The Bulletin of the Cleveland Museum of Art*
Beazley, *JHS 1949*	J. D. Beazley, *The World of the Etruscan Mirror,* in *JHS* 69 (1949) 1–17
Beazley, *EVP*	J. D. Beazley, *Etruscan Vase-Painting,* Oxford, 1947
Beazley-Magi	J. D. Beazley, F. Magi, *La Raccolta Bernardo Guglielmi nel Museo Gregoriano Etrusco,* Vatican City, 1939–1941
Bonfante, *Etr. Dress*	L. Bonfante, *Etruscan Dress,* Baltimore-London, 1975
Bordenache, *Ciste,* I, 1	G. Bordenache Battaglia, *Le Ciste prenestine,* I, 1, Rome, 1979
BullInst	*Bullettino dell'Instituto de Corrispondenza Archeologica*
CII, App.	G. F. Gamurrini, *Appendice al Corpus Inscriptionum Italicarum,* Firenze, 1880
CIL	*Corpus Inscriptionum Latinarum*
Comstock-Vermeule, *Boston Bronzes*	M. Comstock, C. Vermeule, *Greek, Etruscan and Roman Bronzes in the Museum of Fine Arts, Boston,* Greenwich (Conn.), 1971
CSE	*Corpus Speculorum Etruscorum*
de Grummond, *Guide*	N. de Grummond, editor, *A Guide to Etruscan Mirrors,* Tallahassee (Fla.), 1982
De Simone, *Entleh.*	C. De Simone, *Die griechischen Entlehnungen im Etruskischen,* I–II, Wiesbaden, 1968, 1970.
De Ridder, *Bronzes* II	A. De Ridder, *Les bronzes antiques du Louvre,* vol. II, *Les instruments,* Paris, 1913.
DialArch	*Dialoghi di Archeologia*
Ducati, *AE*	P. Ducati, *Storia dell'Arte Etrusca,* Firenze, 1927
Ducati, *RM 1912*	P. Ducati, *Contributo allo studio degli specchi etruschi figurati,* in *RM* 27 (1912) 243–285
EAA	*Enciclopedia del'Arte Antica Classica e Orientale*
EphArch	Ἐφημερίς Ἀρχαιολογική
Fischer-Graf	U. Fischer-Graf, *Spiegelwerkstätten in Vulci,* Berlin, 1980
Foerst, *GPC*	G. Foerst, *Die Gravierungen der pränestinischen Cisten,* Roma, 1978
GazBA	*Gazette des Beaux-Arts*
Gerhard, *ES*	E. Gerhard, *Etruskische Spiegel,* vols. I–IV, Berlin, 1840–1867
GettyMusJ	*The J. Paul Getty Museum Journal*
JHS	*Journal of Hellenic Studies*
Klügmann-Körte, *ES*	A. Klügmann-G. Körte, *Etruskische Spiegel,* vol. V, Berlin, 1897

LAMBRECHTS, *Mir. Mus. Royaux*	R. LAMBRECHTS, *Les miroirs étrusques et prénestins des Musées Royaux d'Art et d'Histoire à Bruxelles,* Bruxelles, 1978	*RA*	*Revue Archéologique*
LIMC	*Lexicon Iconographicum Mythologiae Classicae*	RALLO, *Lasa*	A. RALLO, *Lasa. Iconografia e esegesi,* Firenze, 1974
MANSUELLI, *StEtr 1942*	G. A. MANSUELLI, *Materiali per un supplemento al "corpus" degli specchi etruschi figurati,* in *StEtr* 16 (1942) 531–551	REBUFFAT, *Miroir*	D. REBUFFAT-EMMANUEL, *Le miroir étrusque d'après la Collection du Cabinet des Médailles,* Rome, 1973
MANSUELLI, *StEtr 1943*	G. A. MANSUELLI, *Materiali per un supplemento al "corpus" degli specchi etruschi figurati, II,* in *StEtr* 17 (1943) 487–521	*RendLinc*	*Rendiconti della Accademia Nazionale dei Lincei*
MANSUELLI, *StEtr 1946–47*	G. A. MANSUELLI, *Gli specchi figurati etruschi,* in *StEtr* 19 (1946–47) 9–137	RICHTER, *MMBronzes*	G. M. A. RICHTER, *The Metropolitan Museum of Art. Greek, Etruscan and Roman Bronzes,* New York, 1915
MATTHIES, *PS*	G. MATTHIES, *Die praenestinischen Spiegel,* Strassburg, 1912	*RLouvre*	*La Revue du Louvre et des Musées de France*
MAYER-PROKOP, *Griffspiegel*	I. MAYER-PROKOP, *Die gravierten etruskischen Griffspiegel archaischen Stils,* Heidelberg, 1967	*RM*	*Mitteilungen des Deutschen Archäologischen Instituts, Römische Abteilung*
MEFR	*Mélanges d'Archéologie et d'Histoire de l'École Française de Rome* (vols. 1–82, 1881–1970)	STEINGRÄBER	S. STEINGRÄBER, *Etruskische Möbel,* Rome, 1979
MonAL	*Monumenti Antichi dell'Accademia Nazionale dei Lincei*	*StEtr*	*Studi Etruschi*
MonIst	*Monumenti dell'Instituto di Corrispondenza Archeologica*	*Thes. L.E.I*	*Thesaurus Linguae Etruscae.* I. Indice Lessicale
MonPiot	*Monuments et Mémoires, Fondation E. Piot*		
MusHelv	*Museum Helveticum. Revue suisse pour l'étude de l'Antiquité Classique*		
NS	*Notizie degli Scavi di Antichità*		
NumAntCl	*Numismatica e Antichità Classiche, Quaderni Ticinesi*		
PBSR	*Papers of the British School at Rome*		
PFISTER-ROESGEN, *Spiegel*	G. PFISTER-ROESGEN, *Die etruskischen Spiegel des 5. Jhs. v. Chr.,* Frankfurt, 1975		
PFIFFIG, *Religio*	A. J. PFIFFIG, *Religio etrusca,* Graz, 1975		

OTHER ABBREVIATIONS

B.C.	Before Christ
Biblio. Natl.	Bibliothèque Nationale, Cabinet des Médailles, Paris
ca.	*circa*
cf.	*confer*
cm.	centimeter
D.	Diameter
fig., figs.	figure, figures
gr.	grams
H.	Height
ill.	illustrated
Inv.	Inventory number
L.	Length
Max.	Maximum
n.	note
o.c.	*opere citato*
p., pp.	page, pages
pl., pls.	plate, plates
Pres.	Preserved
s.v.	*sub verbo*
W.	Width

CATALOGUE OF ETRUSCAN MIRRORS AND HANDLES IN MIDWESTERN COLLECTIONS

ANN ARBOR, MICHIGAN

KELSEY MUSEUM OF ARCHAEOLOGY
University of Michigan

1. Engraved mirror. Figs. 1a–d.

Inv. 6714. Provenance: unknown. Purchased from a dealer (in Rome?) before 1911 by Esther B. Van Deman (1862–1937) and willed to the museum in 1938.

Unpublished. For a brief conservation report, see *Research News* (Univ. of Michigan) 23, 5 (Nov. 1972) p. 7. This mirror appears in a short account of Miss Van Deman's collection published by the *Baltimore Evening Sun* on 4 February 1911. A second mirror from the same collection is probably the one now in the Johns Hopkins University Museum, Inv. 9119. It depicts a similar subject.

Bronze. Intact and in excellent condition. Patina: *Obverse,* uneven, light green corrosion products over much of the right half of the disc. This gradually gives way to an area of purple incrustation at the center. Smooth areas of shiny brown and golden bronze appear on the left and lower sections of the disc. The extension and handle have a smooth, dark brown patina covered by irregular patches of dark green corrosion. *Reverse,* the disc surface is rough and pitted. There are a few areas of hard, green and dark brown corrosion, but the overall color is shiny bronze. The handle and extension are smooth and dark brown with patches of dark green corrosion.

Measurements: D., 11.6 cm.; Max. H., 23.8 cm.; L. of handle, 8.0 cm.; W. of extension, 2.8 cm.; W. of terminal, 1.1 cm. Weight, 169.67 gr.

Circular mirror with narrow, concave-sided extension and a handle terminating in a stylized animal head. Disc and handle cast in one piece. The section shows the strong concavity and thin disc typical of later mirrors. The central cavity is deep and resembles a punch mark.

Obverse, a series of deep notches and an enclosing double groove surround the disc and extension. The extension contains the familiar engraved flame motif (*cf.* Nos. **5, 6, 8, 24**) consisting of two leaves from which rise a triangle that in turn supports two curved elements whose interiors are decorated with rows of dots. The stylized flame appears on top. The handle consists of the common configurations of stylized animal (griffin?) heads and a deer-head terminal (see also Nos. **3, 28**).

Reverse, the extension is flat and undecorated except for a pair of deep grooves that echo the concave sides of the extension and continue the plain border of the tondo.

The tondo scene shows two highly stylized figures who face each other in mirror-image juxtaposition. Each wears a Phrygian cap, long hair, and a belted tunic. Simple arcs or vertical lines indicate the drapery folds. In each case the outer arm is bent with hand on hip, but the inner arm is not depicted. The nearer leg is straight; the farther leg is bent at the knee and the foot appears in profile. There is minimal anatomical detail. A small central oval, probably meant to indicate a star, appears between the heads of these figures.

The style is simple, even perfunctory, with no attempt at anatomical accuracy. The engravings, however, are strong, uniform, and confident. There are a few tiny overlappings at the hems of tunics and where legs cross.

This mirror is one of a large class, Mansuelli's "Maestri delle Lase e Dioscuri" (see MANSUELLI, *StEtr 1946–47,* p. 64), which varies only slightly, usually in the treatment of the central "star" or "stars." For a recent discussion of the class, see REBUFFAT, *Miroir,* pp. 483–485. The subject is almost certainly the Dioskouroi. For general discussions of the twin gods and their iconography, see R. DE PUMA in *StEtr* 41 (1973) 159–170; REBUFFAT, *Miroir,* pp. 487–490; R. DE PUMA, *s.v. Dioskouroi, Tinas Cliniar* in *LIMC* III (forthcoming).

We are fortunate to have two excellent parallels for this mirror. The first, Toronto, Royal Ontario Museum 919.26.19 (unpublished), is almost precisely identical in subject, style, measurements, and weight. The Toronto mirror comes from the Bazzichelli Collection, which consisted largely of material excavated in the area around Viterbo. The second is a mirror from Vulci published by U. FERRAGUTI in *StEtr* 11 (1937) 109, fig. 2.

A close, but not precise, parallel comes from a datable

context: Museo Guarnacci 910 from Tomb k at the Portone necropolis near Volterra. Fiumi, who published the mirror in *StEtr* 25 (1957) 384, fig. 13, dated the tomb to two phases: *ca.* 300–280 and 240–230 B.C. Rebuffat, *Miroir,* pp. 578–580, assigns the mirror and the other tomb material to 300–250 B.C.

Another close parallel for the Ann Arbor mirror comes from tomb 5699 in the Monterozzi necropolis at Tarquinia: *NS* 26 (1972) 181, fig. 37, no. 19; p. 182, fig. 38. This mirror is almost identical in size and type but depicts a quincunx rather than one "star" and shows the gods leaning on shields (*cf.* No. **8**). The context suggests a date of 250-200 B.C. Other parallels include Gerhard, *ES* I, pl. 45, 2; Rebuffat, *Miroir,* pl. 25; *CSE* Bologna I, nos. 8, 9, 37; *CSE* Netherlands, no. 2.

About 250 B.C.

2. Engraved mirror. Figs. 2a–d.

Inv. 77.3.3. Provenance: unknown. Given by Mrs. David Dennison in 1977.

Unpublished.

Bronze. The handle, broken off just at the base of the extension, is missing. There is a small crack near the base of the disc. Patina: *Obverse,* very smooth with small surface cracks and some abrasion over entire surface. The disc is a mottled dark brown with lighter green and golden areas, especially on the right side. *Reverse,* similar but not as smooth. Irregular areas of brown and dark green corrosion at edges and especially near bottom of disc. Brown and golden yellow areas at center and top of disc.

Measurements: D., 12 cm.; Pres. H., 15.2 cm.; Handle missing; W. of extension, 2.5 cm. Weight, 119.2 gr.

Circular mirror with narrow, concave-sided extension and handle (now missing) cast in one piece. The section shows the typical concavity of the reverse disc and the char-

acteristic hook-shaped edge with sharp-pointed, triangular profile. There is no central cavity.

Obverse, a series of small beads and an enclosing groove encircle the disc and extension. At the base of the extension are the vestiges of an engraved vegetal motif with additional ornament in punch marks. *Cf.* No. **12** and Biblio. Natl. 1343 in Rebuffat, *Miroir,* pl. 61.

Reverse, the flat extension is decorated with an engraved floral motif. The disc shows a svelte, winged female. She is nude except for a Phrygian cap and shoes. As she strides to the left, wings unfurled but apparently inactive, her head is in profile, but her body is in three-quarter view. She holds her left hand behind her hips and extends her right hand forward to hold a small round object (*cf.* Thorvaldsens Museum no. H2152: T. Melander, *Vᵉ Colloq. Intern. sur les bronzes antiques,* Lausanne, 1978, pl. 99, fig. 10) between her thumb and forefinger.

The design is ample and fills most of the available space on the disc. Compositionally, the subject is simple: the figure's wings form a symmetrical backdrop for the centrally placed vertical of her body. This subject is common, but the quality of the engraving is quite high. Lines are confident, even, and executed in single strokes. There is only one minor overlapping (on the right thigh). One cannot fail to be impressed by the harmonious fluidity of the lines on this simple mirror.

The Ann Arbor mirror belongs to a large class of small hand mirrors with stylized representations of a single striding winged figure, probably a Lasa. Several examples have an archaeological context: (1–2) Tarquinia, Monterozzi necropolis, tomb 5511, nos. 33 and 61 (=*NS* 26 [1972] 191, fig. 47); (3) Tarquinia, tomb 5859, no. 19 (=*NS* 31 [1977] 190, fig. 36); (4) Siena F–20 from the Papena tomb near Siena (=*NS* 21 [1967] 39, fig. 10). The range of dates for these tombs is *ca.* 300–150 B.C., but the mirrors probably belong to the last half of the third century B.C.

About 240–200 B.C.

BLOOMINGTON, INDIANA

INDIANA UNIVERSITY ART MUSEUM

3. Engraved mirror. Figs. 3a–d.

Inv. 62.251. Provenance: unknown. Acquired from Münzen und Medaillen, A. G. (Basel) in 1962.

R. Teitz, *Masterpieces of Etruscan Art* (Worcester 1967), no. 90; pl. 186; L. Bonfante in *GettyMusJ* 8 (1980) 150, n. 18; 153, fig. 11; de Grummond, *Guide*, p. 126, n. 149; *LIMC* II (1984) 943, no. 32.

Bronze. Intact and in excellent condition except for an abraded section of the upper right rim and damaged left point of the extension. Patina: *Obverse,* has been cleaned to produce a hard, smooth surface of black and light green corrosion products. Some areas of shiny bronze, especially near the center. The rim and deep groove surrounding the disc are still encrusted, but the extension and its grooves are smooth. *Reverse,* smooth but flecked throughout with small, light green incrustations making it difficult to read the engravings. Rim is pitted. Lower part of extension and much of handle relief are obscured by corrosion.

Measurements: D., 13.5 cm.; Max. H., 28.4 cm.; L. of handle, 11.6 cm.; W. of extension, 3.2 cm.; W. of terminal, 1.2 cm. Weight, 329 gr.

Circular mirror with concave-sided extension and massive, modelled handle terminating in a stylized ram's head (*cf.* No. **28**.) The disc section shows the raised medallion border and heavy rim profile with deep groove on the obverse typical of the "Kranzspiegelgruppe" (*cf.* Nos. **24, 28, 36**). The edge is undecorated. There is no central cavity.

Obverse, a deep groove surrounds the disc and continues to the points of the extension. Paralleling this on the outside edge is a beaded border. The extension is otherwise undecorated. The handle is elaborately sculpted. A ram's head, with deeply modelled eyes, muzzle, and horns, acts as the terminal. Juxtaposed griffin heads form the central stem; these heads are separated by a striated band. Two acanthus leaves at the top of the handle flare out to the points of the extension. In the V-shaped area between these spreading leaves is a field of numerous punch marks which expands into the extension. The shape of the area covered by these punch marks is roughly that of a concave-sided

diamond. (Compare No. **28**, where this treatment occurs on the reverse.) Mirrors of this type normally have a flame motif filling the extension; it is omitted here.

Reverse, the underside of the ram's-head terminal shows a series of wavy, engraved lines indicating the creature's wool. There is some modelling of the central stem, but this is obscured by corrosion. The acanthus leaves at the top of the handle are not as clearly indicated on this side; between them are the vestiges of another punch-mark area. An engraved acanthus motif fills the extension. This consists of two large, symmetrical leaves with volute bases that open to reveal the tips of three smaller leaves at the top (*cf.* *CSE* Denmark 1, no. 21).

The medallion shows four figures, who occupy the space before an Aeolic façade. At the left an older man sits on a folding stool (*diphros okladias:* Steingräber, type I; p. 332, no. 337). He wears a Phrygian cap and has a himation gathered about his legs and over his left shoulder. He faces right and extends his open right hand toward the other male figure in the scene. A nude woman stands beside the older man. She rests her right elbow on a pillar that is just barely visible behind the seated man. Her jewelry includes a torque, a kestos, and a hair ornament. She is nude but for a large piece of drapery gathered over her left arm, fondled with the fingers of her right hand, and tucked characteristically between her knees. It is not clear whether the foot below the figure belongs to her or to the seated man.

The third figure is a standing youth who faces left. He wears laced sandals, a headband, and a knotted chlamys. He balances a spear almost horizontally on his right shoulder while steadying it with his right hand. Against his left side he holds the severed head of a boar. The fourth figure stands at the extreme right of the medallion and faces left. She wears a belted chiton, hunting boots, and a bracelet on her left wrist. Her hair is neatly arranged in a bun. With her left hand she steadies the handle of a large ax.

Undulating lines at the sides of the medallion indicate a

rocky setting upon which the fourth figure rests her right foot. Some areas behind the figures are shaded by rows of tiny punch marks. For comparable treatments, see GERHARD, *ES* II, pl. 175; III, pl. 276, 4; IV, 284, 2; KLÜGMANN-KÖRTE, *ES,* pls. 82, 2; 87, 1; LAMBRECHTS, *Mir. Mus. Royaux,* nos. 33 and 38. The entire scene is enclosed by a spiky garland with "slide binders" at the four cardinal points. The bottom binder is double (*cf.* No. **24**).

The youthful male figure is identified by inscription on a related mirror (KLÜGMANN-KÖRTE, *ES,* pl. 354, 2) where he again holds a spear and a boar's head. The attributes and the inscription indicate that Meleager (Melacr) is the central figure. For more on the name, see S. DE MARINIS, *s.v. Meliacr* in *EAA* 4 (1961) 987.

The identity of the female nude is more difficult. One would expect Atalanta to appear in a scene with Meleager; but on the inscribed parallel just cited, this figure is called "Arthem," a name that does not correspond to another appearance of Atalanta on a mirror in West Berlin (Fr. 146 = GERHARD, *ES* II, pl. 176; IV, pp. 168–171) where she is labelled "Atlenta." On the Berlin mirror she is nude and sits beside Meliacr (Meleager) but holds a spear. On an uninscribed mirror (GERHARD, *ES* II, pl. 174) she is nude but carries two spears; elsewhere (KLÜGMANN-KÖRTE, *ES,* pl. 94) she is clothed but wields an ax against the Kalydonian boar.

Despite the absence of an inscription, we can easily identify the fourth figure as Vanth by her distinctive costume and attribute. She is labelled on only two mirrors: British Museum 625 (= KLÜGMANN-KÖRTE, *ES,* pl. 110) and Philadelphia, University Museum MS 5444 (= W. N. BATES in *AJA* 15 [1911] 462, fig. 2; *LIMC* II [1984] 343– 344, no. 46). BOARDMAN, in *LIMC* II (1984) 943, no. 32, suggests that this figure may be Artemis. Another mirror (no. 33, once Munich 3654) shows a woman shouldering an ax in the context of another Atalanta-Meleager scene. Boardman tentatively identifies her also as Artemis. But Vanth appears on numerous related objects, especially sculpted cinerary urns, where her iconography is clearly established (see RALLO, *Lasa,* pp. 49–53, for a discussion of the type).

The Indiana mirror is closely related to an example in the Louvre (no. 1041 = GERHARD, *ES* II, pl. 175; DE GRUMMOND, *Guide,* fig. 104). The style, size, and type are almost identical. The subject, except for the figure on the right, is the same: Atalanta with Meleager in the company of the seated Oineos, King of Kalydon. (For similarly posed male figures, see KLÜGMANN-KÖRTE, *ES,* pl. 83, 2 = Louvre 1741.)

The engraving is flexible and confident. There are some overlappings (e.g., Meleager's spear), but these are insignificant. The composition is standard for four-figure groups: seated (or nearly seated) figures flank standing figures before an architectural façade. Meleager's spear effectively connects his head with the King's, although they are on different levels.

About 300–250 B.C.

4. Engraved mirror. Figs. 4a–e.

Inv. 74.23. Provenance: unknown. Acquired in 1974.

Art Journal 34 (1974) 62; BONFANTE, *Etr. Dress,* frontis.; no. 122, pp. 196–197; L. BONFANTE in *StEtr* 45 (1977) 149–168; pls. XXI– XXIII; N. DE GRUMMOND in *Archaeology* 34 (1981) 54 (color photo reversed); DE GRUMMOND, *Guide,* pp. 107, 155–156; figs. 50–51; E. SIMON, *s.v. Althaia* in *LIMC* I, 1, p. 579, no. 1; I, 2, pl. 435, 1; *Guide to the Collections* (Bloomington 1980) p. 44. Inscriptions: *Thes. L. E. I,* pp. 53, 125, 156, 240, 349, 357. *Cf.* DE SIMONE I, pp. 57 (16) and 66 (5).

Bronze. Intact and in excellent condition; a fragment of the tang end is missing. Patina: *Obverse,* a heavy carbonate incrustation covers most of the disc and the tang. The extension has been cleaned to reveal its decorative engravings but these have not been repainted or filled. Other areas of modern mechanical cleaning include the modelled rim and the right edge of the disc. *Reverse,* the entire disc has been carefully cleaned. Previous incrustations were mechanically removed down to a thin layer of red cuprite (especially in the area above Turan's head) and black tenorite. In several areas (e.g., at the base of the extension; near Althaia's left foot; above the horses' heads) the shiny bronze has been revealed. All engraved lines were refilled with a pale green substance, probably a copper carbonate and whiting mixture. Both sides of the mirror were lacquered before acquisition. For more on the condition, see K. J. LINSNER in BONFANTE, *StEtr, o.c.,* p. 168.

Measurements: D., 17.8 cm.; Max. H., 27.5 cm.; L. of extension, 3.5 cm.; W. of extension, 4.1 cm.; L. of tang, 5.7 cm.; Max. W. of tang, 2.1 cm. Weight, 414 gr.

Large circular mirror with concave-sided extension and long, rounded tang. Disc and tang cast in one piece. The disc section shows the gentle concavity and thick rim profile characteristic of this group (see below). The central cavity is carefully cut, hemispherical in section, and about 0.1 cm. in diameter.

Obverse, the disc and extension are surrounded by a deeply modelled ovolo border edged by a simple torus band and a lengthy series of small engraved semicircles. An elaborate engraved palmette decorates the extension; a lyre-shaped pair of volutes encloses the five-petalled palmette.

Reverse, engraved representations fill the disc and extension. At the top of the disc two parallel horizontal lines create an exergue occupied by a central female bust flanked by pairs of horses' heads. The woman, wearing a diadem, pendant earrings, and a bead-and-pendant necklace, is shown in three-quarter view. This is the only figure for whom there is no identifying inscription, but she is most likely Eos (Thesan), the goddess of the dawn, riding in her quadriga. The inner horses face left; the outer two face away from center. Rows of tiny diagonal strokes are used to render highlights on foreheads, cheeks, and eyebrows of these animals. The bridles and bits of each horse are carefully rendered.

There are five large figures in the main frieze. On the left stands Alexandros-Paris. His head, in three-quarter view, faces right. He wears a himation but is barefoot (only the right foot is visible). Tiny diagonal strokes indicate the musculature of his upper chest. A retrograde inscription parallels the long tresses of his wavy hair:

ꟼ⌐ꟼꟼⱯ⊃ꟼꟼ

e l c s n t r e

The second figure, partially obscuring Alexandros, is Athena-Minerva. She stands with her weight resting on her right leg and on the long spear she holds in her left hand. Only the upper portion of the spear is visible beside her face and above her helmet. Her left leg is crossed behind her right and pulls the drapery of her belted chiton between her knees. In addition to the large, crested Corinthian helmet, the goddess wears a pendant earring of undetermined type, a stylized gorgoneion, an armband with four pendant bullae, two bracelets, and sandals. In an uncharacteristic gesture, Minerva places her right wrist against her hip and delicately holds what appears to be a floral bud between her thumb and forefinger. Her name is inscribed retrograde in front of her helmet:

ꟼ⌐ꟼꟼꟼ

m e n r f a

The third figure is Hera-Juno, who stands at the center of the disc facing right, her head in profile. Her hair is drawn up under a twisted fillet. She wears a himation over a thin chiton, a large earring, beaded necklace, armband with four bullae (like Minerva's), two bracelets on her right wrist and one on her left. With her right hand she adjusts the crown on the next figure's head; with her left hand she reaches gently to touch this figure's chin. Her name, inscribed retrograde, appears before her face:

ꟼ⌐ꟼ

u n i

The imposing central figure is seated on a *diphros* with turned legs (STEINGRÄBER, type Ib; p. 332, no. 337a; *cf.* GERHARD, *ES* II, pl. 218 = Biblio. Natl. 1298; LAMBRECHTS, *Mir. Mus. Royaux,* no. 6 = Brussels R 1256). She rests her sandalled feet on a footstool with feet in the shape of animal (lion?) paws (STEINGRÄBER, type 2b). This goddess is Aphrodite-Venus, and her name is clearly inscribed retrograde in the exerque border directly above her head:

ꟼⱯ⌐ꟼꟼ

t u r a n

She wears a chiton and a himation that is elaborately draped over her shoulders and her left arm. Her hair is of medium length, shorter than all of the other figures except Uni's, which is, in any case, gathered up under a fillet. Turan wears an elegant diadem decorated with small square panels, a delicate pendant earring (similar to the one worn by the nude female on No. **14**), a beaded necklace, a larger pendant necklace (*cf.* GERHARD, *ES* II, pl. 212; KLÜGMANN-KÖRTE, *ES,* pls. 27, 49, 60), and a plain bracelet. A long staff or scepter leans on her left shoulder and she holds a mirror in her left hand. The edge of this mirror's disc, as well as the ivory handle with a clearly indicated endpiece, is shown (*cf. CSE* Denmark 1, nos. 4, 24).

The last figure of this major frieze stands at the right and looks toward Turan. Her name, inscribed retrograde, appears above her right arm:

ꟼ⌐ꟼꟼ⊃ꟼ

a l t h a i a

She wears a chiton, a himation wrapped about her arms, and shoes of a type encountered on other fourth-century mirrors (*cf.* Nos. **14, 18–20, 25**). Her jewelry is elaborate: a high crown with nine radiating knobs, a pendant earring, and a beaded necklace. In her right hand she holds a short, leafy (laurel?) branch (*cf.* No. **23**). Her left hand, wrapped in drapery, is placed against her hip in a gesture similar to that used by Minerva.

Two other unusual features appear near the head of this figure. To the right, just at the medallion's edge, is a series of five amorphous curves reminiscent of a stylized Aeolic capital and architrave or perhaps simply a rocky background. I believe the latter interpretation is more likely. Compare Nos. **35, 37,** and KLÜGMANN-KÖRTE, *ES,* pl. 34; see also A. CIASCA, *Il capitello detto eolico in Etruria* (Florence 1962), pl. 24, 1; and N. DE GRUMMOND in *AntK* 25 (1982) 3–14. To the left and directly above Turan's head are four concentric arcs, which appear to hang from the exergue border. A series of small semicircles is attached to the bottoms of alternate arcs. BONFANTE (in *StEtr, o.c.,* p. 152, n. 11) suggests that this motif may represent a parasol and cites a convincing parallel, GERHARD, *ES* IV, pl. 384.

The last figure depicted on this mirror occupies the extension and the lower disc area just above it. His name is inscribed retrograde on the horizontal exergue border immediately above his head:

ꓱ ꓯ ꓦ ꓲ ꓶ

v i l a e

He is a small, nude boy with short, curly hair. He wears the same cross-strapped shoes shown on Althaia's feet plus a necklace with three pendant bullae and an armband with four bullae. He squats on a column base (or altar?) modelled in seven degrees. With his outstretched arms he brandishes two spotted and bearded serpents. The pectorals of this pudgy child are indicated with rows of tiny diagonals like those used on Alexandros and the horses of the upper exergue. Framing the figure of Vilae are scalloped, leaflike elements decorated with small "teardrops."

Uni (Hera) assists Turan while Menrfa (Minerva) and Althaia look on. The scene depicted apparently represents preparations for the Judgment of Paris (Elcsntre). The goddesses behave in an uncompetitive manner. The reason for Althaia's presence is unclear. In Greek mythology Althaia is the daughter of Thestios, sister of Leda, and the mother of Meleager and Deianeira; she is not associated with any of the characters represented on the Indiana mirror. Since this is the only appearance of her name in Etruscan, BONFANTE (*StEtr, o.c.,* p. 152) suggests that "Althaia" may have been confused with "Aithra." This suggestion is further strengthened when we realize that our mirror is closely related to several which show the toilette of Helen, and Aithra is frequently one of Helen's attendants. (See U. KRON, *s.v. Aithra* in *LIMC* I, 1, pp. 425–426.) Without his inscription Vilae (=Iolaos) would surely be identified as the baby Herakles (Hercle) killing the snakes. Here again, the Etrus-

can artist seems to have confused the names of two characters. This time they are related in mythology (Iolaos was Herakles' nephew) rather than in spelling. A figure inscribed "Vile" appears with "Hercle" on a red-figured stamnos, Florence 70528 from Orvieto. See B. ADEMBRI in *Pittura etrusca a Orvieto* (Rome 1982), no. 13, pp. 91–93, with bibliography.

The subject is best understood as a conflation of a toilette scene (the adornment of Turan, Helen, or Malavisch) and the Judgment of Paris. Parallel toilette scenes, especially for the central group of Uni and Turan, appear on GERHARD, *ES* II, pls. 211–216; IV, pls. 383–384; and recently have been studied by D. REBUFFAT-EMMANUEL in *MonPiot* 60 (1976) 53–67 and BONFANTE in *StEtr, o.c.,* pp. 160–166.

The design and quality of engravings on this mirror are excellent. Lines are fluid, sensuous, and drawn in exquisitely controlled single strokes. The delicate use of small rows of tiny diagonals executed with a scorper is an effective contrast to the bold and confident engraved lines. There are no overlappings, but a number of lines are omitted: the back of Menrfa's helmet crest, the back (right) leg of Turan's stool, Turan's right shoulder, the drapery falling from Uni's left hand, Althaia's right shoe, the drapery at Althaia's right shoulder, a torus moulding on the right side of Vilae's base.

The Indiana mirror belongs to a small but very fine group of Hellenistic tang mirrors characterized by their large circular discs (average D., *ca.* 18.8 cm.), heavy rims, pronounced extension points, and long tangs, often with rounded ends. Most are crowded with complex scenes and often have upper and lower exergues, with the quadriga a common subject of the upper. Some good examples in GERHARD, *ES,* include II, pl. 181 (=Biblio. Natl. 1287); pl. 196; III, pl. 257B (=British Museum); IV, pl. 374 (=Amsterdam 1448); pl. 398 (=British Museum 627); pl. 402 (=Leningrad B509); KLÜGMANN-KÖRTE, *ES,* pl. 23 (=Toronto 919.26.30); pl. 34 (=British Museum); pl. 60 (=Florence 72740). Other examples: M. SPRENGER-G. BARTOLONI, *Die Etrusker* (Munich 1980), no. 238 (=Villa Giulia 1745); BONFANTE, *StEtr, o.c.,* pl. XXIV, b (=Florence 84806).

About 300 B.C.

CHICAGO, ILLINOIS

FIELD MUSEUM OF NATURAL HISTORY

5. Engraved mirror. Figs. 5a–d.

Inv. 24376. Provenance: unknown. Purchased in Italy for the museum by Edward E. Ayer in 1895.

R. DE PUMA in *StEtr* 41 (1973) 161–162; fig. 1, b; pl. LII, a–c; R. DE PUMA in *RM* 87 (1980) 26, fig. 9E (disc section).

Bronze. Intact and in fair condition. There is a small crack where disc joins extension. Patina: *Obverse,* chalky, light green incrustations over most of the disc. Two long, parallel abrasions penetrate this layer just below the disc's center. Similar chalky incrustation appears in the recessed areas of extension and handle, but the latter has a smooth, dark green patina, especially above the terminal. A modern metal label has been affixed to the disc. *Reverse,* irregular but smooth patches of light green and dark green patina cover most of the disc. There are minor areas of abrasion at the center and upper disc. Much of the border area and edge of the disc is covered with small, irregular patches of incrustation and dirt. The handle and extension have a relatively smooth, uniform, dark green patina.

Measurements: D., 13.6 cm.; Max. H., 29.1 cm.; L. of handle, 12.0 cm.; W. of extension, 3.4 cm.; W. top of handle, 1.9 cm.; W. of terminal, 1.5 cm. Weight, 249 gr.

Standard grip mirror with circular disc, concave-sided extension, and a handle terminating in a deer's head. Disc and handle cast in one piece. The section shows the characteristic features of this type: a heavy, undecorated edge with small hook on the obverse and sharp triangular profile on the reverse, a gentle concavity on the reverse, and a thick, clearly defined disc border. The central cavity is round in section and 0.14 cm. in diameter.

Obverse, the unengraved disc is surrounded by a beaded border, which continues down the sides of the extension. The extension is filled with a typical flame motif (*cf.* Nos. **1, 6, 8, 24, 27, 28**). In this case the flame rises from two elements that are decorated with small, parallel horizontals. They 'are flanked by single rows of small punch marks. The three leaves below these motifs are enlivened with tiny punched dots. The central stem of the handle shows two opposed animal heads, perhaps griffins. Details

of the relief are picked out with small engraved lines. The terminal is in the shape of a deer's head, with engraved curves indicating hair and striated ears.

Reverse, a simple cable pattern frames the medallion. The extension is embellished with a cursory lotus bud design (*cf.* Nos. **2, 22, 24, 28**), while below, at the top of the handle, are a series of small punch marks. The underside of the deer-head terminal is engraved with numerous small, wavy lines to indicate skin.

Four figures occupy the medallion. On the left and right, facing each other, are nearly identical males, who wear Phrygian caps, long tunics belted across the chest, and laced sandals. Each stands with his outer arm held behind his back and with legs crossed; the inner arms are invisible. Perhaps these figures are meant to be leaning against the short Ionic pillars at the edge of the medallion. Wavy groundlines rise up the sides of the disc between them and the cable border.

Two more figures are represented between these flanking males. On the right a nude female with long, wavy hair stands in a position frequently encountered on mirrors with four-figure compositions (*cf.* Nos. **6, 24, 33**; see also Nos. **27, 36**). She wears laced sandals and has drapery tucked between her thighs. Behind her and to the left is another female, who stands with right arm extended to embrace or touch the male who stands to the left. This second woman wears a Phrygian cap and long chiton. A small pediment, unsupported by columns, floats above the heads of the four figures.

Mirrors with the same configuration of four figures are quite common but not always easy to identify with certainty. The flanking male figures are almost surely the Dioskouroi, Castur and Pultuce. In fact, they are so identified by inscriptions on some related mirrors: GERHARD, *ES* I, pl. 59, 3 and III, pl. 268 (=Brussels R 1272; LAMBRECHTS, *Mir. Mus. Royaux,* no. 22). Other inscribed mirrors assign different names to these same figures (e.g., GERHARD, *ES* I, pl. 59, 2 = Villa Giulia 24894, where they are Aplu and Laran). In the case of the rather homogeneous four-figure mirrors presented in this fascicle (Nos. **5, 6, 24, 33**), the flanking males are likely to be the twin deities because of their costumes and the architectural elements (vestigial dokana?) shown with them.

The clothed woman is most likely interpreted as Minerva, and she is so indentified by inscription or attributes on a number of mirrors of this group (e.g., GERHARD, *ES* III, pl. 255 B). The nude woman is more difficult to identify. One thinks of Helen in connection with her brothers, and this figure, when inscribed, is identified as Helen on some examples (e.g., New York, Metropolitan 21.88.27; KLÜGMANN-KÖRTE, *ES,* pl. 84, 2). But she is also identified as Turan (GERHARD, *ES* III, pl. 257 C), Thalna (Brussels R 1288 = LAMBRECHTS, *Mir. Mus. Royaux,* no. 38), or Uni (KLÜGMANN-KÖRTE, *ES,* pl. 84, 1) on other mirrors. For more on this problem, see R. DE PUMA, *o.c.,* pp. 167–168; REBUFFAT, *Miroir,* pp. 462–469.

The mirror represents a popular design. Compositionally, the arrangement of figures is simple: two very similar males heraldically flank two females who turn their attention to the outer figures. The engraving is reasonably firm and uniform but not particularly flexible. There are several overlappings and some omissions.

Stylistically, the Chicago mirror seems to be a debased version of a mirror published by K. D. MYLONAS in *EphArch* (1883) 249–254, pl. 13. Other parallels include Louvre 1784 = GERHARD, *ES* III, pl. 266, 2; pl. 277, 4; KLÜGMANN-KÖRTE, *ES,* pl. 84, 1. All of these, and many more, illustrate the peculiar omission of engraved lines under the right arm of the nude central figure (*cf.* No. **33**).

Late third or early second century B.C.

6. Engraved mirror. Figs. 6a–d.

Inv. 105170. Provenance: unknown. Purchased in Italy for the museum by Edward E. Ayer in 1895.

R. DE PUMA in *StEtr* 41 (1973) 162–163; fig. l, c; pl. LIII, a–c.

Bronze. Intact and in good condition. Patina: *Obverse,* the lower half of the disc is covered with a rough, dark brown incrustation, but above, much of the shiny bronze is visible. This upper area is marred by a series of vertical striations and scratches. The handle

and extension have a uniform, smooth, dark brown patina. *Reverse,* smooth, dark brown patina over the disc, extension, and handle. Heavy pitting in the border and at bottom and left of medallion. Parts of the upper rim are also chipped or pitted.

Measurements: D., 12.6 cm.; Max. H., 25.6 cm.; L. of handle, 10.1 cm.; W. of extension, 3.4 cm.; W. top of handle, 1.7 cm.; W. of terminal, 1.4 cm. Weight, 319 gr.

Standard grip mirror with circular disc, concave-sided extension, and a handle terminating in a deer's head. Disc and handle cast in one piece. The section shows the characteristic features of this type: a heavy, undecorated edge with small hook on the obverse and triangular profile on the reverse, a gentle concavity on the reverse, and a thick, clearly defined disc border. There is no central cavity.

Obverse, the reflecting disc is surrounded by a deep groove and beaded border, which continue to the points of the extension. A standard flame motif occupies the extension (*cf.* Nos. **1, 5, 27**); a series of dots surrounds the motif. The handle presents the usual deer-head terminal surmounted by juxtaposed griffin (?) heads and modelled acanthus leaves at the base of the extension.

Reverse, a garland of olive (or laurel) leaves frames the medallion. A simple engraved "X" fills the extension; below it random dots occupy the surface between the modelled acanthus leaves. Some curved lines mark the underside of the terminal.

The subject and composition of the four-figure scene on the medallion is identical to No. **5**. A minor difference is the omission of rocky groundlines at base and sides. Stylistically, the figures are even more abstracted than on No. **5**; this is especially noted in the rendering of the female nude. However, drapery may be said to be slightly more realistic than the depiction on No. **5**.

The engraving is uniform, flexible, and very confident. There is much fluidity in the lines of the figures and the leafy border. There are relatively few overlappings, but there is some sloppiness in the details of the figures' heads and hats. A good parallel for the style and subject is a mirror from the Tomba dei Calinii Sepuś near Monteriggioni, now in the Bianchi Bandinelli Museum at Colle Val d'Elsa (see M. MARTELLI, *Prospettiva* 5 [April 1976] 71, fig. 2). Material in this tomb runs from the late fourth to early first century B.C. Other parallels, especially for the treatment of the nude figure's hair, include two examples in the Bibliothèque Nationale: REBUFFAT, *Miroir,* pls. 69–70.

Second century B.C.

ORIENTAL INSTITUTE
University of Chicago

The six Etruscan mirrors and fragments in the Oriental Institute (Nos. **7–12**) are part of a much larger group of Etruscan bronzes collected by a Mayor Luciardi, apparently near the end of the last century. (One early label suggests a date of 1889 for one piece.) The collection was sold by A. Rambaldi, a Bolognese antiquities dealer, to Ira Nelson Morris either in 1913 (when President Wilson appointed Morris commissioner general to Italy) or at some point between the World Wars. Morris died in 1942; his widow gave the entire collection to the Oriental Institute in 1947.

7. Engraved mirror. Figs. 7a–d.

Ira Nelson Morris Study Collection, no. 1076. Provenance: unknown. Given by Constance Rothschild Morris in 1947.

Unpublished.

Bronze. Intact but heavily corroded and with some deep cracks along the edge of the disc. Patina: *Obverse,* large areas of heavy, powdery, light green incrustation on left and right sides of the disc. The center and top are smoother with only shallow layers of azurite deposits. The tang is covered with bright green incrustations on each edge. *Reverse,* hard, heavy incrustation layers over entire surface of disc but with smoother levels on extension. Tang is heavily corroded with a light green product.

Measurements: D., 13.2 cm.; Max. H., 18.4 cm.; W. of extension, 2.2 cm.; L. of tang, 3.8 cm. Weight, 161.9 gr.

Piriform mirror with rounded extension and long, pointed tang. Disc and tang cast in one piece. The section shows the very slight curvature and thickening at the edge typical of early mirrors. (*Cf. CSE* Bologna I, nos. 25, 26, 28.) There is no central cavity.

Obverse, a beaded border surrounds the disc and extension. An engraved palmette consisting of nine fronds decorates the extension and lower disc. A pair of elegant volutes flanks the palmette. Reverse, undecorated.

Two close parallels for the decoration and shape of this mirror appear in *CSE* Bologna I, nos. 26 and 28; the latter is also especially close in size and disc section. Another parallel is in the Vatican: Beazley-Magi, pl. 53, no. 13; p. 186.

Late fifth to middle fourth century B.C.

8. Engraved mirror. Figs. 8a–d.

Ira Nelson Morris Study Collection, no. 3370. Provenance: unknown. Given by Constance Rothschild Morris in 1947. See No. **7.**

Unpublished.

Bronze. The handle is broken off at the base of the extension. The disc and extension are relatively well preserved. There is a shallow dent on the obverse disc. Much of the reverse disc is abraded. Patina: *Obverse,* smooth, hard layers of azurite, especially at the top and edges of the disc plus the extension. Brown and light green patina covers the lower half of the disc. *Reverse,* similar to obverse but with more azurite areas and some patches of a matt, dark brown patina.

Measurements: D., 11.1 cm.; Pres. L., 13.5 cm.; W. of extension, 2.4 cm.; Pres. L. of extension, 2.4 cm. Weight, 163.3 gr.

Circular mirror with concave-sided extension and, originally, a handle terminating in a stylized animal head. Disc and handle cast in one piece. The section shows the pronounced concavity and thin disc characteristic of later mirrors. The central cavity is 0.2 cm. in diameter.

Obverse, the decorative format is identical to No. **1.** For other mirrors with this motif, see Nos. **1, 5, 6, 10, 24, 27, 28, 33, 34,** and **36.** Remnants of the tips of acanthus leaves at the base of the extension indicate that the handle's design was also like that of No. **1.**

Reverse, a plain shelf borders the medallion and con-

tinues down the sides of an undecorated extension (*cf.* No.
1). The medallion shows two highly stylized males, who
wear simple knee-length tunics belted high above the waist.
They also wear Phrygian caps; sandals or boots are not
indicated. Each figure leans backward against a large shield
rendered in profile. Between them, at the level of their
waists, are three horizontal lines, perhaps representing the
dokana (*cf.* No. **22**). Precisely between the figures' heads is
a large "star" consisting of a small circle from which radiate
four large and four small petal-shaped elements.

The style is very close to No. **1**. The engravings express
a confidence gained by repetition. There are a few minor
overlappings. For the subject the Dioskouroi, see discussion
for No. **1**. Other close parallels include Toronto 919.26.20
(= DE GRUMMOND, *Guide,* figs. 56–57), which is virtually
identical in subject and size; Toronto 919.26.21 (unpublished); New York, Metropolitan 831 (= RICHTER,
MMBronzes, pp. 484–485); Brussels R 1290 (= LAM-
BRECHTS, *Mir. Mus. Royaux,* no. 40); *CSE* Bologna I, nos.
8–9; Yale University Art Gallery no. 1952.52.8 (unpublished); Volterra, Guarnacci 910 (= *StEtr* 25 [1957] 384,
fig. 13); Viterbo 402/998 (= A. EMILIOZZI, *Coll. Rossi
Danielli,* no. 589; pp. 256–257; pl. 189).

About 250 B.C.

9. Fragmentary engraved mirror. Figs. 9a–d.

Ira Nelson Morris Study Collection, no. 5439. Provenance:
unknown. Given by Constance Rothschild Morris in 1947.
See No. **7.**

Unpublished.

Bronze. In 1983 the mirror was recomposed from twenty-six sur-
viving fragments. Approximately 14 percent of the disc is lost. The
lacunae have been filled and inpainted. The handle terminal is
missing. Patina: *Obverse,* areas of smooth, blue and light green
corrosion cover most of the disc. The perimeter shows a rougher,
warty incrustation. Repaired gaps have been inpainted with light
green. *Reverse,* the surface has been cleaned down to the cuprite
level and, in some areas, to the shiny bronze. The central disc is
mostly a maroon-colored area of smoothed warts.

Measurements: D., 12.2 cm.; Max. Pres. H., 22.6 cm.; W. of
extension, 3.1 cm. Pres. Weight, 111.5 gr.

Circular mirror with concave-sided extension and a
handle that originally ended in a stylized animal head. Disc
and handle cast in one piece. The disc section shows the
gentle concavity and triangular edge profile with small indentation typical of many mirrors (*cf.* Nos. **5, 6, 27, 33, 37**
for intact examples). A central cavity is not visible.

Obverse, the decorative format for the disc is similar to
No. **5**: a beaded border and parallel, shallow channel, which
continue to the tips of the extension. No engraved ornament
is visible on the extension. Vestiges of three modelled leaves
appear at the top of the handle. Their bases are bound by a
crosshatched band. A deep central groove runs down the
spine of the handle. The remains of a beaded ornament also
appear on either side.

Reverse, no ornament is visible on the extension. Three
leaves, comparable to those on the obverse but better preserved, decorate the top of the handle. The other elements
(crosshatched binder, central groove, beaded edge) are identical to those on the obverse.

The heavy corrosion layers make it impossible to see
but a few elements of the original design. A simple cable
pattern once framed the medallion; this is now visible only
at the upper left, top, center right, and lower right and left
portions of the border. The best-preserved element of the
figural scene is a large, symmetrical plant, which occupies
the lower center of the disc but grows upward to the disc's
middle. This plant once consisted of nine large fronds. Portions of what is most likely a large star appear directly
above the central plant (*cf.* Nos. **8, 22**), and above this are
the vestiges of a pedimental construction (*cf.* Nos. **5, 6**).

A few additional elements are barely discernible. These
consist of several graceful lines, which generally follow diagonal patterns to either side of the central plant. These are
no doubt the vestiges of drapery lines covering the bodies of
two symmetrically disposed figures. A few crossed lines
near the base of the left figure may indicate sandal straps.
Some additional curves behind each figure seem to depict
the lines of two shields shown in profile (*cf.* No. **8**).

It seems clear that only two figures are represented.
Their symmetrical position and their clothing (drapery, sandals), as well as the iconographic clues (shields, star, pediment), corroborate their identification as the Dioskouroi.
Centrally placed plants are also frequently associated with
these twin deities. The Oriental Institute example is particularly close to GERHARD, *ES* I, pl. 47, 1 (= Berlin Fr. 94),
which shows a plant plus the cable pattern, shields, and
pediment. Other examples with plants flanked by the
Dioskouroi include GERHARD, *ES* I, pl. 46, 9; pl. 48, 4–5
(= Berlin Fr. 97 and 87); LAMBRECHTS, *Mir. Mus. Royaux,*
nos. 44–45, 71 (= Brussels R 1293–R 1294, A 3140); *StEtr*
25 (1957) 384, fig. 14 (= Volterra 907); *CSE* Netherlands,
no. 14; Louvre Br. 1792; Florence, Museo Arch. 635.

Compositionally, the mirror represents a type frequently encountered: nearly identical figures flank a series

of attributes placed in a vertical sequence between them. No. **22** is close both in composition and style.

About 300–250 B.C.

10. Fragmentary engraved mirror. Figs. 10a–d.

Ira Nelson Morris Study Collection, uninventoried. Provenance: unknown. Given by Constance Rothschild Morris in 1947. See No. **7.**

Unpublished.

Bronze. Only the central portion of the very thin (*ca.* 0.75 mm.) disc is preserved. There are several small cracks at the edge of this fragment. The second fragment preserves the base of the disc and the extension. The handle is missing. Patina: *Obverse,* a smooth brown layer has flaked off exposing a powdery, light green corrosion on the disc. The extension fragment is smooth and a uniform gray-green color. *Reverse,* a fine, uniform, light green patina covers most of the disc and upper extension. There are large patches of a brown-yellow corrosion at the edges.

Measurements: Disc fragment Max. W., 8.6 cm.; Max. H., 9.4 cm. Extension fragment Max. W., 5.1 cm.; Max. H., 5.6 cm. Pres. H. of fragments joined, 13.3 cm. Pres. Weight, 51.3 gr.

Circular mirror with concave-sided extension and, originally, a handle terminating in a stylized animal head. Disc and handle cast in one piece. The section shows a graceful concavity. Small sections of the edge, preserved on the extension fragment, indicate that the edge profile was of standard type (*cf. CSE* Bologna I, no. 11; LAMBRECHTS, *Mir. Mus. Royaux,* no. 51). There is no central cavity.

Obverse, small notches enliven the raised edge of the extension and once circumscribed the disc. A shallow channel parallels the edge. The extension ornament is an engraved flame motif similar to Nos. **1, 5, 6, 8, 24, 27, 28, 33, 34,** and **36** but more debased than usual.

Reverse, there are no indications of extension ornaments or borders. The disc shows a nude, winged figure standing to the left, with right leg tense and left leg relaxed. The upper portion of the profile head is missing, but a small arc on the nape of the neck suggests that the figure once wore a Phrygian cap (*cf.* No. **2**). The figure's right hand is held behind the hip; the right arm and hand hang lifelessly at the side. Anatomical renderings are slight: a flowing line down the chest and abdomen, small male genitals. There are no indications of breasts, knees, or toes.

The design is simple and familiar. The unfurled wings help to frame the figure while expanding to fit the medallion shape (*cf.* Nos. **2, 18**). The engravings are steady and fluid.

There are minor overlappings (the tip of the right foot) and places where lines fail to connect.

The figure is clearly a member of the popular race of Lasae so frequently depicted on Etruscan mirrors (Nos. **2, 18, 19**), but here the Lasa is clearly male. Stylistically, the mirror is close to No. **2** and other members of the large group of mirrors with a single Lasa shown striding to the left. Lasae standing, rather than striding, are less common. Examples, both male and female, are GERHARD, *ES* I, pl. 31, 4–5; pl. 32, 5–7; LAMBRECHTS, *Mir. Mus. Royaux,* nos. 50–51 (= Brussels R 1299–R 1300); REBUFFAT, *Miroir,* pl. 58 (= Biblio. Natl. 1340); *cf. CSE* Denmark 1, no. 19. For discussion of the chronology, see No. **2.**

About 250–200 B.C.

11. Fragmentary unengraved mirror. Figs. 11a–b.

Ira Nelson Morris Study Collection, uninventoried. Provenance: unknown. Given by Constance Rothschild Morris in 1947. See No. **7.**

Unpublished.

Bronze. The mirror consists of eighteen fragments with a major lacuna above the attachment of the tang. Most of the fragments were glued to a cardboard mount before acquisition. Due to the fragility of the pieces, it has not been possible to remove them from the mount. Figs. 11a–b show only the reverse side of the object. Individual fragments that can be lifted and examined reveal no traces of engraved ornament on the obverse. Patina: *Obverse,* the pieces that can be examined show corrosion products identical to those on the reverse. *Reverse,* large areas of powdery, light green corrosion cover most of the fragments. Where this has flaked off, a level of dark green patina is exposed. Patches of dark brown indicate areas that were in recent contact with an oily substance of undetermined type.

Measurements: D., 15.1 cm.; Max. H., *ca.* 18.5 cm.; L. of tang, 3.1 cm.; Max. W. of tang, 1.2 cm. Pres. Weight, *ca.* 142 gr.

Slightly ovoid mirror with separately attached tang. The disc section shows a slight thickening at the edge and a characteristic triangular profile (*cf. CSE* Bologna II, no. 8). There is no discernible concavity and no central cavity. The tang consists of two elements joined to the disc with three rivets. The first element is a thin, fan-shaped disc with a handle, the edges of which are folded back and rounded. The second element, on the reverse, is another fan-shaped disc of identical type and size but without a handle. These two semicircular plates fit over the edge of the mirror and are joined to it by three rivets (*cf. CSE* Bologna II, nos. 21–22; MAYER-PROKOP, *Griffspiegel,* pl. 35, 1).

Probably early fifth century B.C.

12. Mirror handle. Figs. 12a–d.

Ira Nelson Morris Study Collection, uninventoried. Provenance: unknown. Given by Constance Rothschild Morris in 1947. See No. **7.**

Unpublished.

Bronze. The handle, extension, and a small portion of the lower disc are preserved. Heavy corrosion obscures much of the modelled detail. Patina: *Obverse,* heavily encrusted with dark green and powdery, light green patches. *Reverse,* corrosion deposits are lighter.

Measurements: Pres. L., 14.5 cm.; W. of extension, 2.8 cm.; L. of handle, 8.2 cm.; W. of terminal, 0.9 cm. Weight, 37.3 gr.

Mirror handle terminating in an animal head; originally cast in one piece with a circular disc mirror.

Obverse, the disc was originally surrounded by a deep groove and a notched border, which now frame the extension. A deeply engraved floral motif decorated the extension. The handle stem shows vestiges of paired leaves and deep crossbands. It terminates in a modelled ram's head.

Reverse, the extension is undecorated and no remains of engraved lines are visible on the small disc area that survives. The underside of the handle is undecorated but shows the deep notches of the crossbands flanking a vertical furrow.

Although fragmentary, this handle is easily identified as coming from a common type of circular mirror represented here by No. **2.** Other examples include *CSE* Denmark 1, no. 19; Biblio. Natl. 1343 (= REBUFFAT, *Miroir,* pl. 61); *CSE* Netherlands, no. 17; *CSE* Bologna I, nos. 3 and 33; *cf. CSE* Bologna I, nos. 31 and 32, where this floral motif is combined with the more popular flame motif. It is likely that the missing disc was originally engraved with a winged figure.

Third century B.C.

CLEVELAND, OHIO

CLEVELAND MUSEUM OF ART

13. Engraved mirror. Figs. 13a–d.

Inv. 16.2012. Provenance: unknown. Purchased for the museum by Harold Parsons. Gift of the John Huntington Art and Polytechnic Trust in 1916.

R. D. DE PUMA in *RM* 87 (1980) 26–27, fig. 9D (disc section); R. D. DE PUMA in *BClevMus* 70 (1983) 295–296, figs. 13–15.

Bronze. A small lucuna and long crack at top of disc. Patina: *Obverse,* heavily encrusted eruptions, especially on the lower two-thirds of the disc. A broad band about 10 cm. long at upper left and center of disc has been polished to reveal a light green patina. There are small areas of azurite in the extension. The handle is better preserved and has a strong, even green patina. *Reverse,* a smooth green patina with areas of dark green, bright intense green, and small red patches. A number of small areas are pitted. There is evidence of some mechanical abrasion visible under magnification. Corrosion makes the incisions very difficult to read, but the quality of the line is strong and firm. The central cavity is 0.3 cm. in diameter, hemispherical in section, and almost 0.1 cm. deep.

Measurements: Horizontal D., 18.8 cm.; Vertical D., 22.5 cm.; Max. H., 36.1 cm.; H. of handle, 11.8 cm.; W. of extension, 4.2 cm.; W. top of handle, 2.3 cm.; W. of animal terminal, 1.4 cm. Weight, 488 gr.

Large piriform mirror having an extension with concave sides and a handle terminating in a stylized deer's head; disc and handle cast in one piece. The flat edge is decorated with an ovolo relief about 0.6 cm. high. The section is slightly convex, with the hooked profile of the edges frequently found on Praenestine mirrors.

Obverse, a shallow groove surrounds the disc and extension. The handle is modelled with beaded borders that flank a long, flat central rib. This rib terminates in the modelled deer's head at the base and in a semicircular area with a leafy-scallop design at the top. (The leafy-scallop design is similar to that on No. **20**). Above these shallow relief leaves

are the poorly preserved remains of an incised floral ornament consisting of a lyre-shaped palmette, tendrils, and blossoms.

Reverse, the handle is concave and undecorated. An incised olive or laurel leaf border rises from the extension to frame the entire disc and surround the two female figures. Both women wear long chitons, bracelets, and cross-strapped shoes. The one on the left also has a mantle draped about her right arm and across her waist; she wears an elaborate earring. Both figures are shown in profile and face each other as if conversing. The right figure holds a long spear in her right hand. The spear's point pierces the leaf border at the top of the disc. A crescent occupies the space between her right hand and the head of the left woman. A number of vegetal forms, including tendrils, blossoms, and a grapelike cluster, fill the space behind the spear-bearing woman. An unidentified object appears in the heavily corroded area beneath the right arm of the left woman.

The only clues to the identity of these figures are the crescent and spear. If, indeed, these are attributes, we may tentatively suggest that the mirror depicts Artemis and Athena conversing. On Etruscan mirrors Athena is usually shown with a full complement of attributes (see No. **20**), but she appears on at least two mirrors with only a spear: KLÜGMANN-KÖRTE, *ES,* pls. 63, 2, and 67, where she is positively identified by inscription. The figure of Losna (Luna) on Villa Giulia 24864 (GERHARD, *ES* II, pl. 171) bears a long staff and faces a crescent. For related mirrors, *cf. ES* IV, pls. 310–311.

The piriform shape, characteristic disc section, and stylistic features (like the way in which the figures overlap the leafy border) associate this mirror with Praenestine workshops. For the obverse handle treatment, compare Brussels R 1269 and R 1279 (see LAMBRECHTS, *Mir. Mus. Royaux,* no. 19, pp. 121–123; no. 29, pp. 181–183). The engraving style of the latter is similar to that of the Cleveland mirror.

About 330–300 B.C.

14. Engraved mirror. Figs. 14a–e.

Inv. 20.170. Provenance: unknown. Purchased by Harold Parsons from A. Barsanti (dealer) in Rome. Given by Mrs. John Huntington in 1920.

R. D. De Puma in *RM* 87 (1980) 5–28, figs. 1–4; 9C; pl. 3; R. M. Gais, *s.v. Aigithos* in *LIMC* I, p. 378, no. 49; R. D. De Puma in *BClevMus* 70 (1983) 296–301, figs. 17–21.

Bronze. A section of the rim (reverse, right side indicated by hatching on Fig. 14a) approximately 9 cm. long is restored. This, however, does not affect the incised design on the reverse. Patina: *Obverse,* uneven, spotted dark green and yellow-brown patches. In upper left and central disc area are patches of maroon-colored shiny bronze. Handle is not encrusted but smooth and dark green. The terminal is split and heavily corroded. *Reverse,* smooth but of uneven color; areas of light and dark green, plus some brown with much speckling, over entire disc. Handle is brown and dark green. The central cavity is 0.23 cm. in diameter, hemispherical in section, and fairly shallow.

Measurements: Horizontal D., 17.5 cm.; Vertical D., 20 cm.; Max. H., 32.9 cm.; H. of handle, 11.6 cm.; W. of extension, 3.8 cm.; W. top of handle, 2.3 cm.; W. of animal terminal, 1.5 cm. Weight, 418 gr.

Piriform mirror having an extension with concave sides and a handle terminating in a stylized deer's head; disc and handle cast in one piece. The flat edge is decorated with an ovolo relief about 0.5 cm. high. The section is slightly convex.

Obverse, a shallow groove surrounds the disc and extension and continues down the sides of the handle to the base of the deer-head terminal. The handle is modelled with three convex reliefs, two of which flare out at the top into the points of the extension. The third relief, centrally placed, remains straight but blossoms into two acanthus leaves in the extension. Above these relief leaves are the vestiges of an engraved floral ornament, probably a palmette. Reverse, the handle is concave and undecorated. On the extension is a poorly preserved inverted palmette flanked by small volutes. Two branches of a large olive or laurel tendril rise from this area to form the disc border. A large four-petalled flower closes the border at the top of the disc. In the triangular area at the base of the disc above the extension is a large four-petalled rosette with four fernlike leaves and a single tendril. See De Puma, *o.c.,* pp. 9–10, fig. 4, for discussion and parallels for the vegetal ornament.

The figured scene consists of four characters. At the center a powerful nude male with curly hair and beard strides to the right. The top of a scabbard appears below his left arm; its strap is slung across his right shoulder. In his right hand he carries a sword, which he uses to threaten a young boy he holds precariously in his left arm. The boy is

nude save for a bulla, bracelets, and an anklet. A tendrilled plant springs incongruously from his right shoulder. A nude young female stands to the left of this central group and appears to restrain the bearded man with both hands. Her hair is crowned with a leafy wreath; she wears an elaborate necklace, pendant earring, an anklet, cross-strapped shoes, and some fluttering drapery decorated with tiny tassels. All three nude figures are characterized by anatomical details rendered with short curving strokes. The fourth figure is an old woman, who kneels at the right. She has dishevelled short hair and wears a simple peplos and some bands on her left arm.

The figures stand on a series of groundlines rising to the right. Some stylized tendrils grow from this: one, between the man's legs, has a large bell-shaped flower; a second appears in front of the kneeling old woman. A large acorn-shaped plant with five large leaves and a flowing tendril floats between the heads of the nude man and woman. Behind the woman is another tendril; it supports a large grapelike cluster of blossoms.

The engravings are shallow and fine, but the quality is delicate and sure. A number of minor "errors" occur. For a complete discussion, see De Puma, *o.c.,* pp. 23–24.

The scene represented on this Praenestine mirror is probably Telephos holding the young Orestes hostage. The old woman on the right would then represent the boy's nurse. Often, but not always, depictions of this subject in Etruscan art show Telephos and Orestes at an altar. Frequently, the parents of Orestes, Clytemnestra and Agamemnon, are also present. The nude young woman on this mirror is not likely to represent Clytemnestra but may depict a Lasa who attempts to protect the child from harm. For a lengthy discussion of the iconography, see De Puma, *o.c.,* pp. 11–22.

Other mirrors with the subject are Louvre 1729 (Klügmann-Körte, *ES,* pl. 142, where the figures are inscribed Lycurgos, Taseos, and Pilonikos, the son of Taseos) and an example from the Tomba dei Calinii Sepuś near Monteriggioni (Bianchi Bandinelli in *StEtr* 2 [1928] 160–161, no. 172; pl. 34; De Puma, *o.c.,* pp. 20–21, fig. 7). The Monteriggioni mirror is now in a Swiss private collection.

The piriform shape, the characteristic disc section, and especially the style of engraving indicate that this mirror is Praenestine. The closest parallel is Paris, Biblio. Natl. 1323 (Rebuffat, *Miroir,* pp. 214–219, 494–498; pl. 41–72; *cf.* De Puma, *o.c.,* pp. 27–28) excavated at Praeneste. For the obverse rim and handle treatment, compare Bologna It. 733 (*CSE* Bologna I, no. 4) and Brussels R 1262 (Lambrechts,

Mir. Mus. Royaux, no. 12, pp. 86–87). For the figure style, compare a cista in Berlin: BORDENACHE, *Ciste,* I, 1, pl. LVI, 4a.

About 330–300 B.C.

15. Engraved mirror. Figs. 15a–f.

Inv. 52.259. Provenance: unknown. Purchased through the J. H. Wade Fund from B. Tartaglia (dealer) in Rome in 1952.

S. E. LEE in *BClevMus* 40 (1953) 32–34; MAYER-PROKOP, *Griffspiegel,* no. S 14, pp. 19, 64–67; pls. 13, 1; 53, 6 (rim detail); O. VON VACANO in *Gnomon* 43 (1971) 295–296; PFISTER-ROESGEN, *Spiegel,* pp. 112, 130; H. JUCKER in G. KOPCKE and M. MOORE, eds., *Studies in Classical Art and Archaeology: A Tribute to P. H. von Blanckenhagen* (Locust Valley, N.J., 1979), pp. 53–54; pl. 15, 1 (drawing after cleaning); R. DE PUMA in *RM* 87 (1980) 26, fig. 9B (disc section); FISCHER-GRAF, p. 12, n. 122; DE GRUMMOND, *Guide,* pp. 141–143; fig. 83 (drawing before cleaning); R. DE PUMA in *BClevMus* 70 (1983) 290–295; figs. 1–5.

Bronze. Completely preserved except for a small section of the lower right (obverse) rim. Patina: *Obverse,* very smooth, fine, light blue-green patina over entire surface. A small abraded area at top right reveals the shiny bronze. A series of twelve small, circular incrustations on tang and lower disc; a large eruption at top of disc plus another damaged area on the left edge. Museum accession number applied in red paint. *Reverse,* similar to obverse. Smooth, light green patina with vague patches of shiny bronze revealed by recent cleaning. Several areas of heavy, dark brown corrosion in upper left quadrant of disc. The shape of one of these areas is roughly a quatrefoil; three smaller areas form the points of a triangle surrounding the "quatrefoil." This configuration suggests that another metal object had lain upon the mirror for a long period. Some tiny surface cracks near the center of the disc.

Measurements: D., 15.2 cm.; Max. H., 19.9 cm.; H. of tang, 3.2 cm.; W. of extension, 3.3 cm.; W. of tang, 1.2–1.5 cm. Weight, 546.5 gr.

Mirror with small extension and short, slightly tapered tang. The disc section has a very shallow convexity. The thick edge (0.6 cm.) is decorated with an elaborate ovolo and beaded border separated by a plain torus moulding. There is no central cavity.

Obverse, unengraved. The delicate beaded border surrounds the disc but is worn smooth near the extension.

Reverse, the edge is slightly raised and offset. The border is engraved with a continuous ivy wreath whose inner and outer leaves point in opposite directions. The figured scene depicts a winged female, who carries the body of an armed warrior in her arms. Both faces are in profile. Hair is indicated by wavy lines. Small almond-shaped eyes, arcs for

eyebrows, and volutes for ears complete the faces. The female has four elaborately detailed wings, which symmetrically frame her large body. She flies to the left, but her head faces right to look at the warrior's face. She wears a pointed diadem, a necklace, a chiton, billowing mantle, and large, winged shoes. The hems of her garments are decorated with rows of small punched dots. Her right hand clutches the warrior's left thigh; her left hand cradles his hip.

The warrior's right arm is draped over the female's back so that his hand touches her right shoulder. His left arm, both legs, and his head hang free to indicate that he is dead. He wears a chitoniskos, the lower hems of which are again decorated with dots, a cuirass, and greaves. The carefully rendered cuirass is ornamented with a meander and zigzag across the chest and two bands of paired verticals alternating with dots across the belly. Shoulder flaps and pteryges are also visible. Arcs decorate the greaves and are probably stylized indications of the muscles they protect. A crested Corinthian helmet, fallen from the warrior's head, appears beneath the figures. A scalloped line ornaments the crown; the crest has a row of dots topped by a series of nine small squares that support paired vertical lines.

Incisions are deep and approximately 0.025 to 0.03 cm. wide. In most areas they are consistent and sure. A punch was used to form single rows of dots decorating Eos' crown, her neck and breast, the hems of her garments, the hem of Memnon's chitoniskos, and his helmet. Irregularly spaced dots appear on Eos' wings and winged shoes.

For the subject Eos carrying the body of her son, Memnon, see A. MINTO in *MonAL* 28 (1922) cols. 254–288; MAYER-PROKOP, *Griffspiegel,* pp. 64–67; FISCHER-GRAF, pp. 12–14; JUCKER, *o.c.; CSE* Denmark 1, no. 22. For other representations of Eos with four wings, see MAYER-PROKOP, *Griffspiegel,* S 12, 47, 52. For similar depictions of armor, see New York, Metropolitan 22.139.84 (=FISCHER-GRAF, V 15). Also see BORDENACHE, *Ciste* I, 1, pls. XVII, VIIb; XXIV, IXa–b; CXXVIII, 26b. For similar style and border motif, see Copenhagen, Thorvaldsens Museum 156 (=MAYER-PROKOP, *Griffspiegel,* S 15). Compare for similar drapery style and use of dots: Berlin, Collection Dorow 572, and Vienna VI 2627 (=MAYER-PROKOP, *Griffspiegel,* S 7 and S 10). Other parallels include Brussels R 1270 (=LAMBRECHTS, *Mir. Mus. Royaux,* no. 20); Villa Giulia 18038 (=MAYER-PROKOP, *Griffspiegel,* S 48); Bologna It. 746 (=*CSE* Bologna I, no. 10). The disc section is closely paralleled by a mirror in a Bern private collection: I. JUCKER in *MusHelv* 39 (1982) 5–14, fig. 3. For similar weight and section, compare *CSE* Denmark I, nos. 2 and 26.

LEE, *o.c.,* p. 33, dated this mirror to the first half of the fourth century B.C. He believed it was archaizing rather than archaic. Mayer-Prokop, *Griffspiegel,* p. 66, n. 200, rightly disputed this date as too late. She associated the style with that of an unspecified dancer depicted in the Tomb of the Triclinium and thus implied a date in the early fifth century B.C. Pfister-Roesgen, *Spiegel,* p. 112, agreed with this conclusion but offered a more specific range, the first quarter of the fifth century B.C. De Grummond, *Guide,* p. 143, assigned the mirror to *ca.* 460 B.C.

About 470–460 B.C.

Doubts concerning the authenticity of the engravings on Cleveland 52.259 were voiced by O. von Vacano, *o.c.,* in a review article of Mayer-Prokop's monograph. Ulrike Fischer-Graf, *o.c.,* only mentions the Cleveland mirror in passing, but H. Jucker (*o.c.,* p. 53, n. 3) reports that she also questions its antiquity. It should be noted that, to the best of my knowledge, neither von Vacano nor Fischer-Graf has examined the mirror in person. Their conclusions were apparently based on photographs made before the object was cleaned in 1976. This brief review will first consider some of the stylistic objections voiced by von Vacano and then report on recent microscopic investigations of the patina.

The mirror presents several unusual stylistic features. Perhaps the most atypical is the ivy leaf border on the reverse. Most mirrors have border designs that rise in opposite directions from the tang or base of the disc; some device, often a knot or blossom on Vulcian mirrors, terminates their juncture at the top of the disc. On the Cleveland mirror the border is continuous; in addition, the inner leaves point clockwise, while the outer leaves point counterclockwise.

Other early mirrors have continuous ivy leaf borders: Munich 3971 (=Pfister-Roesgen, *Spiegel,* S 3); Copenhagen, Thorvaldsens Museum 156 (=Mayer-Prokop, *Griffspiegel,* S 15); London 540 (=S 28); Villa Giulia 18005 (=S 53). Other devices, including continuous anthemia, chevrons, guilloches, and wave crests, appear on many other mirrors, showing that continuous borders, as such, are not rare. The position of the leaves, pointing in opposite directions, is unusual but not unique: London 546 from Chiusi (=Klügmann-Körte, *ES,* pl. 14; Mayer-Pro-

kop, S 38, which is also like the Cleveland example in that it has no obverse ornament). One may note that such alternating ivy borders also occur on painted pottery (e.g., P. Ducati, *Pontische Vasen,* pls. 22–23). Jucker, *o.c.,* p. 54, noticed the interesting correspondence between the number of ivy leaves on the inner border of this mirror and the Vatican relief mirror with Eos and Kephalos (Pfister-Roesgen, *Spiegel,* S 2). The same number, 35 leaves, also occurs on another stylistically related mirror in Copenhagen (Mayer-Prokop, *Griffspiegel,* S 15).

The unusual placement of the dead warrior's helmet at the bottom of the disc has aroused suspicion. On other versions of this subject on mirrors, Memnon's helmet is either absent or he still wears it. The artist of the Cleveland mirror apparently wished to convey the speed with which Eos carries off her son. There is no time to retrieve his helmet; it remains as a symbol of the chaos of the battlefield. A very similar use of a helmet appears at the base of a tondo on a fragmentary Attic white-ground plate from the Acropolis (B. Graef and E. Langlotz, *Die antiken Vasen von der Akropolis zu Athen* II, 1933, pl. 32, no. 425; *cf.* J. Neils in *AntK* 23 [1980] 19, no. 54; p. 21).

Several of von Vacano's concerns about Eos' garments and Memnon's armor are now, after cleaning, less troublesome. For example, the "necklace" around Eos' neck (Fig. 15e) is now more likely interpreted as part of her mantle. A hem with meander border and a smaller necklace of dots has appeared beneath the corrosion. Similarly, the flaps of Memnon's cuirass are now visible and clearly make more sense.

In 1983 I personally examined the mirror with a good binocular microscope. It was clear that a light green patina covered all areas of engraving and that malachite crystals had grown over several engraved lines. Smaller crystals appeared within individual channels. Several of the dots punctuating the hems of Eos' garments are crossed by tiny surface fissures. Numerous engraved lines disappear under the large, hard brown incrustations. Of course, the corrosion products removed earlier had obscured several engraved areas (Figs. 15e–f). These examinations indicate that the engravings on the mirror are ancient, however unusual (at the present state of our knowledge) specific stylistic features may appear.

COLUMBIA, MISSOURI

MUSEUM OF ART AND ARCHAEOLOGY
University of Missouri

16. Bone handle. Figs. 16a–k.

Inv. 63.18. Provenance: unknown. Acquired in 1963.

F. Cummings in *The Missouri Alumnus,* March 1964, p. 7, fig. 14; J. D. Cooney in *BClevMus* 55 (1968) 263, fig. 4; S. Weinberg in *Muse, Annual of the Museum of Art and Archaeology* 9 (1975) 25–33; figs. 1–3.

Bone. Portions of the cylindrical surface are smooth and well preserved (Figs. 16a, b, d–g), but other areas are abraded, so that much of the relief design is lost (Figs. 16h–j). The cylinder is a thin-walled tube (0.3 to 0.8 cm. thick) without the soft cellular interior of a new bone fragment. There is a small hole directly behind the younger female's head at the top of her wing (Figs. 16a, d, k). The lower section of the cylinder is missing. Presumably, this once had a plain border like the one preserved at the top.

Weinberg, *o.c.,* p. 33, n. 2, reports that this object was examined by Dr. B. M. Gilbert of the University of Missouri Anthropology Department. Dr. Gilbert identified the bone as section of the (right?) femur of a common ox or cow (*Bos sp.*) and noted the existence of a natural hole for the nutrient foramen, a blood vessel (Figs. 16c, k, to the left of the younger woman's right wrist).

This handle is particularly interesting because it preserves several vestiges of paint and gilding (*cf.* Y. Huls, *Ivoires d'Étrurie,* Brussels, 1957, p. 177). The background was painted a dark blue (a strong patch is visible under the young woman's chin, Figs. 16d–e); red touches appear on the young female's lips, the upper feathers of all four wings, and portions of the crouching youths at the bottom of the handle. Gilding is preserved on the wings (in many places it occurs over or near the red paint), the objects the women carry, and their leafy crowns (Fig. 16k).

Measurements: Max. D., 4.85 cm.; Pres. H., 10 cm.; H. of top border, 0.5 cm.; Max. Depth of reliefs, *ca.* 0.7 cm.

Cylindrical bone handle for a tang mirror. For carved handles in general, see Huls, *o.c.,* nos. 111–118, pls. 49–53; Gerhard, *ES* I, pl. 54, 2–3; III, p. 49; Weinberg, *o.c.; CSE* Denmark 1, nos. 4, 12, 24; *CSE* Bologna II, no. 4. For an ivory handle of similar type and style in a German private collection, see *Kunst der Etrusker* (Hamburg 1981) no. 117.

The carved frieze on the Missouri handle shows two pairs of figures (Fig. 16k). There are two winged females, who occupy almost the entire height of the cylinder and who move to the left in nearly identical fashion. Each wears a fillet or crown with leaflike appendages (*cf.* Gerhard, *ES* II, pl. 122, female head depicted in mirror extension, and pl. 294 for similar crowns), perhaps meant to indicate a wreath, and a belted chiton with sleeves almost reaching the elbow. Drapery is elegantly rendered; the overfolds billow sensuously and anatomical features are visible beneath the lower portions of the chitons. The profile faces have long noses, almond-shaped eyes, and heavy lips; one female appears younger (Figs. 16a, d) than the other (Figs. 16b, g).

Between the wing tips of each female are the vestiges of smaller crouching figures. The better preserved of these figures (Fig. 16j) sits on the ground with the right arm bent at the elbow and extended across the chest. The figure's left arm, which may have rested on its leg, is extended toward the feet of the younger female (*cf.* Gerhard, *ES* I, pl. 29, 17). The figures are too abraded to determine sex or specific details of action. It is likely that they are male children. We may compare some similarly posed children on mirror extensions and on a pair of ivory appliqués, tentatively identified as prisoners, previously on the Basel art market (see *Münzen und Medaillen, Sonderliste O* for December 1972, p. 22, nos. 58b–c; *cf.* Weinberg, *o.c.,* p. 33, n. 27).

The specific subject is difficult to determine. Weinberg, *o.c.,* p. 32, tentatively suggests connections with the cult of Aphrodite. Any attributes the children may have held are now missing. The female figures, with their large wings, chitons, and crowns, fit the iconography for Lasae. The objects they hold delicately between their fingers may offer a further clue. These appear to be flexible, sausage-shaped bags. Winged figures hold similar objects on a number of mirrors: Gerhard, *ES* I, pl. 34, 3; II, pl. 143; Klügmann-Körte, *ES,* pls. 16; 22; *cf.* p. 214, for a mirror with a seated youth holding a similar object identified as a diadem. These objects are usually identified as folded fillets offered to visible or invisible recipients. It is unlikely that the Lasae are presenting the fillets to the children because the fillets are held too high; the connection between the winged women and the seated children remains tenuous.

Late fourth century B.C.

17. Engraved mirror. Figs. 17a–d.

Inv. 80.191. Provenance: unknown. Purchased from Edward Merrin Gallery, New York, in 1980.

GazBA 97 (March 1981) p. 26, no. 142; M. Del Chiaro in *Muse, Annual of the Museum of Art and Archaeology* 15 (1981) 54–57; O. Overby, ed., *Illustrated Museum Handbook, A Guide to the Collections in the Museum of Art and Archaeology* (1982) no. 83; de Grummond, *Guide,* fig. 107.

Bronze. Generally in excellent condition. The tang is friable, its patina abraded, and a portion of its base missing. A small crack penetrates the disc near the edge at the three o'clock position on the reverse. Patina: *Obverse,* uneven green patina with much of the surface pitted, especially near the center and upper right quadrant of disc. Extension is a darker green and relatively smooth. The beaded border along the edge is considerably worn. *Reverse,* smooth, even, light green patina. There are areas of pitting near the heads of both figures, above Hermes' left shoulder, across Herakles' right foot and near his right shin, across his left shin, and around the central cavity. There are also minor scratches and small gouged areas. The area about Herakles' left biceps appears to be a modern refill.

The central cavity is irregularly shaped. At time of acquisition this was filled with green wax. Upon removal of the wax it was noted that the cavity is unpatinated and, as it now stands, is probably not ancient.

Measurements: D., 16.6 cm.; Max. H., 22.8 cm.; L. of tang, 4.0 cm.; W. of extension, 4.2 cm. Weight, 390.5 gr.

Circular tang mirror with concave-sided extension. The slightly convex edge is undecorated. The section is convex with a gradual thickening at the edge but without indentation or hook on the obverse (*cf. CSE* Bologna I, nos. 26, 28, 40).

Obverse, the vestiges of a beaded border, once surrounding the disc and extension, are best seen along the edge of the extension. Poorly preserved engraved volutes flank a small palmette on the extension (*cf.* Biblio. Natl. 1285 = Rebuffat, *Miroir,* pl. 3, obverse).

Reverse, two nude males, identified by their attributes, face each other on the medallion. At the left is Herakles (Etruscan Hercle), who wears his lion skin over his shoulders, its forepaws knotted beneath his neck. The lion's head is the hero's cap. His right hand holds the end of the gnarled club, which rests on the disc's border. His left foot rests atop a large amphora. There is a large bird perched on Herakles' right shoulder (*cf.* Gerhard, *ES* II, pl. 156).

At the right is Hermes (Turms), recognizable by his winged petasos and the caduceus (the distinctive finial is visible above his hat) held in his right hand. He wears a long chlamys. The figures stare directly into each other's eyes and stand in an awkward posture more suited to sitting or leaning against an object. Behind each figure is a bizarre plant consisting of a stylized acanthus leaf from which sprouts a long stalk with a small round flower at its tip (*cf.* Brussels R 1263 and A 383 = Lambrechts, *Mir. Mus. Royaux,* nos. 13, 67).

The border is an elaborate branch whose thick stalks bear alternating leaves and berry clusters. It springs from a pair of delicate volutes that enclose a palmette with seven fronds above and a large lotus bud below. At the top of the disc the ivy stalks are knotted together. The ivy stalk border is closely paralleled by Brussels R 1263; the extension motif is very similar to those on Cambridge GR.12.1864 (= Gerhard, *ES* II, pl. 178; Fischer-Graf, V69) and Toronto 919.26.31 (= Klügmann-Körte, *ES,* pl. 56; Fischer-Graf, V61).

The engraving is smooth, confident, and even, especially in the contours of the figures and the ivy border.

The subject and composition associate this mirror with five others: (1) Naples 5567 (= Gerhard, *ES* II, pl. 129; Fischer-Graf, V73); (2) Once Rome, Collegio Romano (= Gerhard, *ES* II, pl. 130; Fischer-Graf, V92); (3) Biblio. Natl. 1285 (= Rebuffat, *Miroir,* pl. 3; Fischer-Graf, V82); (4) Perugia 998 (= Gerhard, *ES* II, pl. 128; Fischer-Graf, V88); (5) Boston 97.2740 (= Comstock-Vermeule, *Boston Bronzes,* no. 377). For two additional mirrors with parallel representations of Herakles, see Klügmann-Körte, *ES,* pls. 63, 2, and 64. There are other objects with three-figure compositions whose outer figures parallel the two representations of the Missouri mirror: Bologna It. 1072 (= *CSE* Bologna I, no. 12) and Biblio. Natl. 1288 (= Gerhard, *ES* II, pl. 154; Rebuffat, *Miroir,* pl. 6). See also the bronze reliefs above the feet of the Ficoroni Cista: T. Dohrn, *Die Ficoronische Ciste,* Berlin 1972, pl. 27.

Late fourth or early third century B.C.

18. Engraved mirror. Figs. 18a–d.

Inv. 83.224. Provenance: unknown. Acquired by Dr. and Mrs. Robert Waelder in 1959; gift of Mr. and Mrs. Cedric Marks, 1983.

D. G. MITTEN-S. DOERINGER, *Master Bronzes from the Classical World* (Mainz 1967), no. 215; R. DE PUMA in *Muse, Annual of the Museum of Art and Archaeology* 20 (1986), forthcoming.

Bronze. Two portions of the disc are modern restorations indicated by stippling on Fig. 18a. Engravings in these areas are modern attempts to approximate the original designs. The thin disc is cracked at the base near the extension. Three modern cloth patches of rectangular shape have been added to the obverse. Patina: *Obverse,* original areas are covered by a dark green-brown patina with numerous irregular pits of various sizes. The modern copper restorations have been painted to match the original surface. *Reverse,* much of the original patina has been covered by modern paint carefully spattered to create a smooth, mottled surface, especially on the right side.

Measurements: D., 15.2 cm.; Max. H., 22.2 cm.; L. of tang, 4.2 cm.; W. of tang, 1.1 cm.; W. of extension, 2.6 cm. Weight, 97.3 gr.

Circular mirror with concave-sided extension and long tang with a rounded base. Mirrors from Vetulonia and Orvieto, now in Florence, have nearly identical shapes (see D. LEVI in *StEtr* 5 [1931] 519–521, pl. 25, and *Pittura etrusca a Orvieto,* Rome 1982, no. 17, pp. 97–98). The central cavity is a shallow circle approximately 0.1 cm. in diameter. The section is very thin, slightly convex, and with characteristic thickening at the edges (*cf.* LAMBRECHTS, *Mir. Mus. Royaux,* no. 54).

Obverse, there is no engraved decoration. A worn, but still visible, notched border surrounds the disc and extension; a similar, but more mechanical, border has been provided for the modern restoration.

Reverse, a large, winged nude female moves to the left in the characteristic cross-step pose. Her voluminous unfurled wings expand to fill most of the medallion. She wears a large pendant earring, a necklace of beads, an arm bracelet with three pendants (almost surely meant to be bullae), and shoes. She holds a large alabastron awkwardly in her left hand (*cf.* No. **19**) and balances a perfume dipstick on the fingers of her right hand. Her elegant face is shown in profile; the coiffure is elaborate and encloses what appears to be a fillet or diadem (*cf.* the similar headresses on GERHARD, *ES* I, pl. 112). The pose is similar to that of the nude warrior on No. **25** and to the more abstract figure on No. **2**.

A winged Lasa, identified as such by inscription, is shown on two mirrors with her alabastron and dipstick. A famous example in the Bibliothèque National (no. 1287 = REBUFFAT, *Miroir,* pp. 51–64; pls. 5 and 71; RALLO, *Lasa,* no. 13) illustrates two Lasae carrying these attributes. It is probable that the winged female on the Missouri mirror is also a Lasa (see DE PUMA, *o.c.,* forthcoming).

The robust design effectively fills the medallion. The Lasa's form extends along the disc's vertical axis into the extension. The flowing contours of her body are echoed in the undulating lines of the wings, which flank and frame it. In most areas the lines are engraved with a fluid, confident touch. Some hesitancy may be noted in the rendering of the hair. There are minor overlappings where dipstick meets forearm and where the fingers of the left hand grasp the alabastron. The lower left leg from the knee down appears to be retraced. There are several faint lines engraved along the sole of the left shoe. The Lasa's knee, her left wing tips, and the odd base of the alabastron are modern engravings. The appearance of the engravings, before restoration, may be seen in MITTEN-DOERINGER, *o.c.*

This mirror stands near the beginning of a large group showing flying Lasae. Most, like our No. **2**, are far more stylized. Some parallels for the Missouri mirror include *CSE* Denmark 1, nos. 12, 16, and 23; *CSE* Netherlands, no. 22; *CSE* Bologna I, no. 30; *NS* 26 (1972) 162, no. 40; 31 (1977) 169, no. 10; LAMBRECHTS, *Mir. Mus. Royaux,* nos. 52 and 54. A series of unpublished examples in the Royal Ontario Museum, Toronto, is also close (nos. 919.26.4 through 919.26.7). See also S. MASTRANDER in *Serta Eitremiana* (1942) p. 102, fig. 1; *Münzen und Medaillen, Sonderliste T* (Oct. 1981), no. 99.

Probably 300–275 B.C.

CRAWFORDSVILLE, INDIANA

WABASH COLLEGE ANTIQUITIES COLLECTION

19. Engraved mirror. Figs. 19a–e.

Inv. 94. Provenance: unknown. Purchased in Rome by members of the Elston Family in 1909.

Unpublished.

Bronze. Very thin disc with three lacunae (*ca.* 0.4, 1.6, and 3.3 cm. across) and several cracks, many of which follow the engraved lines of the reverse. The tang is missing. Patina: *Obverse,* very fine noble patina of light green. Some darker discolorations caused by encrusted dirt and oils. Numerous tiny surface cracks near the edges. Fine scratches, uniformly distributed, are the result of modern cleaning. There is an overall pitting, which is especially concentrated near the right edge. *Reverse,* smooth, uniform, light green patina. Fine scratches resulting from mechanical cleaning over much of the surface. Shallow pitting over upper portions of left and central figures. Encrusted dirt at lower left and around disc's perimeter. Two rivets (*ca.* 0.6 cm. in diameter) hold a broken handle to the extension. This covers the engraved floral ornament.

Measurements: D., 17.2 cm.; Max. H., 20.4 cm.; L. of extension, 3.3 cm.; W. of extension, 2.7 cm.; L. of riveted handle, 4 cm. Weight, 169.83 gr.

Circular bronze mirror with extension and missing tang replaced by a riveted fragmentary handle. The flat edge, 0.4 cm. wide, is unornamented. The section is convex with a relatively thick edge (*cf. CSE* Bologna I, no. 2). There is no central cavity.

Obverse, a wide but shallow groove surrounds the disc and extension. At the edge, vestiges of a continuous row of dots, now much worn. Engraved ornaments on the extension and lower disc depict a large palmette of seven fronds flanked by acanthus leaves. The palmette springs from a series of three rings that are obscured by two rivets holding the handle fragment on the opposite side.

Reverse, on the extension is a large palmette with seven fronds flanked by elegant flowers. The palmette rises from a leaflike form only partially visible to the left of the riveted handle. Above, on a single groundline, stand three winged females. The largest, at the center, wears a belted chiton fastened with round buttons or knots at the shoulders. She also wears a pointed diadem, a pendant earring, beaded necklace, arm bracelets, and cross-strapped shoes. The arm bracelets, worn just above the elbow by all three figures, find close parallels on several mirrors (e.g., GERHARD, *ES* II, pls. 183, 200, 201, 204; III, pl. 270, 2; KLÜGMANN-KÖRTE, *ES,* pl. 17) and on Etruscan red-figure vases of the Clusium Group (see M. HARARI, *Il "Gruppo Clusium" della ceramografia etrusca* [Rome 1980], pls. III, 1; VIII, 1; IX, 2; X, 1; XXI, 2; XXVII, 1–2). She holds an alabastron in her extended left hand and a flower (a bud on a stem, apparently) in her lowered right hand. She looks to the right, where a smaller sister, dressed identically, approaches with left hand raised in salutation. She grasps a larger alabastron in her left hand. Rising from the groundline between these two figures is a bizarre volute, perhaps meant to indicate a fanciful plant (*cf.* Boston 13.2888 = COMSTOCK-VERMEULE, *Boston Bronzes,* no. 395). Between their heads are two stars: one consists of four circles and four petal-like elements radiating from a central circle; the other is obscured by a layer of encrusted dirt but now consists of two radiating "petals."

The third figure is partially nude. She holds the end of a piece of billowing drapery in her left hand while gathering a knot of it between her legs. The gesture is familiar from many other mirrors: GERHARD, *ES* I, pl. 84; II, pls. 149; 203; 206; 207, 4; 230; 231; III, pls. 262, 2; 271A, 1; 244, 1; 275A, 2–3; 276, 3–4; 277, 2–7; 278, 2–6; 279, 1; 280; IV, pls. 290; 300, 1–2; 323; 341, 1; 351, 1–3; 374; KLÜGMANN-KÖRTE, *ES,* pls. 79; 80, 2; 81, 1; 84, 1–2; 85, 1–2. In her right hand she holds the same kind of flower as the central figure does (*cf.* GERHARD, *ES* II, pl. 212). All three women wear their hair in the same distinctive manner: a row of four large, circular curls in front of the diadem and a triangular cluster of three curls at the back above the nape. For a close parallel for this coiffure, see GERHARD, *ES* I, pl. 95, and II, pl. 165.

The elegant dress, coiffure, and jewelry, plus of course, the wings and alabastra, suggest that these three females are Etruscan Lasae. For Lasae carrying alabastra, see No. **18**, and RALLO, *Lasa,* pp. 48–49. The subject and style are paralleled by a number of mirrors: GERHARD, *ES* III, pls. 271A, 1; 248, 2; IV, pl. 315A. Brussels R 1296 (=KLÜG-MANN-KÖRTE, *ES,* pl. 17; LAMBRECHTS, *Mir. Mus. Royaux,* no. 47) is close. Examples with similar palmettes and floral motifs are GERHARD, *ES* I, pl. 69; II, pl. 201; IV, pl. 298; KLÜGMANN-KÖRTE, *ES,* p. 213; *CSE* Bologna I, nos. 13 and 38; COMSTOCK-VERMEULE, *Boston Bronzes,* no. 395. The composition and several iconographical details are paralleled by a mirror from Toscanella, now Florence 77759: MANSUELLI, *StEtr 1942,* 539–540; pl. XLIII, 2.

Engraved lines are firm, uniform, and flowing; they are deep considering the thinness of the disc (0.05 cm. near the center).

About 300–275 B.C.

DAYTON, OHIO

DAYTON ART INSTITUTE

20. Engraved mirror. Figs. 20a–d.

Inv. 70.34. Provenance: unknown. Purchased from the André Emmerich Gallery, New York, in 1970 with funds provided by the Zimmerman Foundation.

Art of Ancient Italy (Emmerich Gallery, New York, 1970), no. 19, p. 13; M. DEL CHIARO, *Re-exhumed Etruscan Bronzes* (Santa Barbara, 1981), no. 26, p. 31; *LIMC* II (1984) 1062, no. 162.

Bronze. Intact and in excellent condition. Patina: *Obverse,* powdery, light green areas near base of disc, darker green and brown over remaining areas. The handle is very dark green with some white incrustations in the grooves. *Reverse,* bright green patina and incrustations near edge of disc, especially at bottom. A dull blue-green corrosion is mixed with patches of dirt over the laurel leaf border. The central disc is a smooth, dark brown with scattered patches of green. There are heavy, dark green incrustations on the handle.

Measurements: Horizontal D., 17.5 cm.; Vertical D., 18.8 cm.; Max. H., 33 cm.; H. of handle, 12.5 cm.; W. of extension, 4.4 cm.; W. top of handle, 2.6 cm.; W. of animal terminal, 1.4 cm. Weight, 514.7 gr.

Piriform mirror having an extension with concave sides and pronounced points and a handle terminating in a stylized deer's head with carefully modelled features. Disc and handle cast in one piece. The rounded edge is decorated with a small beaded border that surmounts a frieze of vertical flutes about 0.7 cm. high. The section shows the characteristic curvature and hook of Praenestine mirrors and has a distinctive flat edge (*cf.* Brussels R 1262 = LAMBRECHTS, *Mir. Mus. Royaux,* no. 12). The central cavity is round (0.3 cm. in diameter) and deep.

Obverse, a deep groove creates a sharply defined border around disc and extension. The delicate beaded border continues down the sides of the handle but stops at the base of the animal terminal (*cf.* No. **39**). Two parallel ridges flare upward toward the extension and end as the edges of a fanlike element in relief at the base of the extension. For similar treatments of this area, see No. **13** and also MATTHIES, *PS,* pl. 1, or LAMBRECHTS, *Mir. Mus. Royaux,* no. 12.

The engraved designs at the base of the disc are poorly preserved. They consist of a symmetrical arrangement of acanthus leaves, a central palmette, and pairs of volutes with stylized flowers.

Reverse, the handle is concave and undecorated. A typical olive leaf garland frames the disc. At irregular intervals small berry clusters appear. A large trumpet-shaped flower grows from the base of this framing garland, while a starlike flower appears at its top. Three large figures occupy the disc. On the left Minerva stands with most of her normal attributes. She wears a helmet, the aegis, and a decorated peplos; she carries a spear in her right hand and a shield, whose interior is ornamented with a wave-crest pattern, on her left arm. In addition, she wears elegant pendant earrings, bracelets, and cross-strapped shoes. A small owl hovers above her shield.

At the center a nude female faces right to offer a beribboned laurel leaf crown to the third figure, a seated male. The woman has long hair tied with a ribbon. Like Minerva, she wears pendant earrings, bracelets, and shoes. Some drapery falls from her left upper arm. Behind her is a small dog, who offers Minerva a leafy tendril he grasps in his mouth.

The male, seated on a rock at the right, is nude but for the himation gathered across his lap. With his right hand he steadies a beribboned thyrsos against his thigh. Delicate arcs delineate the anatomical features of the two nudes. The engraver was particularly attentive to the rendering of hair (*cf.* No. **14**). In each case the iris and pupil of the eye are indicated by a single vertical stroke; this is true even for the tiny eyes of the gorgoneion on Minerva's aegis. For a parallel of this treatment of eyes, see British Museum 719 from Palestrina (=KLÜGMANN-KÖRTE, *ES,* pl. 120). The nude couple is clearly Dionysiac and perhaps represents Ariadne and Dionysos.

The figures form a simple, pleasing composition with the nude female placed along the central axis of the disc and paralleled by the vertical figure of Minerva on the left. Typically for mirrors associated with Praeneste, the medallion is crowded with details and the figures extend into the leafy border. Engraved lines are firm yet delicate. There are several overlappings, notably in connection with Minerva's spear and shield strap.

The distinctive shape, size, section, and engraving style of this mirror mark it as a product of a Praenestine workshop (*cf.* Nos. **13, 14, 21, 23, 38, 39**). For a similar Minerva, see GERHARD, *ES* II, pl. 191, and KLÜGMANN-KÖRTE, *ES,* pl. 55. The unusual dog is paralleled on GERHARD, *ES* III, pl. 248A; IV, pls. 311 and 389 (= British Museum 623). For closely related border motifs, see GERHARD, *ES* IV, pl. 328, and KLÜGMANN-KÖRTE, *ES,* pl. 20.

Late fourth century B.C.

DETROIT, MICHIGAN

DETROIT INSTITUTE OF ARTS

21. Engraved mirror. Figs. 21a–d.

Inv. 47.399. Provenance: unknown. Formerly in the collection of Sir Guy Francis Laking, London. Acquired from E. S. David (Long Island City, New York) in 1947 with funds from the Founders Society, the Laura H. Murphy Fund.

Christie's *Sale Catalogue* for 19 April 1920, no. 4; Spink and Son, Ltd., advertisement in the *Burlington Magazine* for May 1920; F. W. ROBINSON in *Bulletin of the Detroit Institute of Arts* 27, 3 (1948) 67–68; DE GRUMMOND, *Guide,* p. 66; figs. 7, 64; R. DE PUMA in *Atti del Secondo Congresso Internazionale Etrusco* (Florence 1986), forthcoming.

Bronze. Intact and in excellent condition. Patina: *Obverse,* most of the surface is smooth and shiny. It varies in color from dark brown-green to light golden brown. There are major areas of dark, rough corrosion on the upper right edge, lower center and left of the disc. Incrustation is heaviest in the groove on the left side of the disc. The handle is smooth, worn along the edge, and has a golden patina except for the animal terminal, which is brown and has traces of white and light green corrosion. The edge is well preserved, with only traces of dark green incrustation. *Reverse,* smooth except for some rough areas along the right edge beyond the engraved border. Several patches of bright green patina, especially on the lower half of the disc. Some areas appear to have been cleaned and smoothed in recent times. The handle is a smooth, golden brown with only minor traces of bright green patina.

Measurements: Horizontal D., 17.5 cm.; Vertical D., 18.0 cm.; Max. H., 30.6 cm.; H. of handle, 12.3 cm.; W. of extension, 3.8 cm.; W. top of handle, 1.6 cm.; W. of animal terminal, 1.2 cm. Weight, 470.9 gr.

Piriform mirror with a short extension and a handle terminating in a stylized deer's head. The disc and handle cast in one piece. The flat edge is decorated with an ovolo border (*cf.* LAMBRECHTS, *Mir. Mus. Royaux,* no. 6, p. 48 = Brussels R 1256). The section has the characteristic hook and rounded profile associated with mirrors from Praeneste (*cf.* Nos. **13, 14, 20, 23, 38, 39**). There is no central cavity.

Obverse, a beaded border and shallow groove surround the disc, extension, and handle, ending at the deer-head terminal. The central spine of the handle is flat with a rounded top projecting into the extension. A large palmette is engraved above this. It consists of nine fronds with two single stalks of berries flanking the central frond. The base has two volutes from which spring symmetrical leafy tendrils. Small punch marks decorate the lower portion of the extension. Small dots also decorate the top of the deer-head terminal. The transitional area between the deer's neck and the handle is incised with short arcs.

Reverse, the handle is flat, smooth, and undecorated except for the terminal, which has a small curved line marking the underside of the deer's head. On the extension a cluster of five large acanthus leaves surrounds a trumpet-shaped flower. Directly above this are the seven fronds of a partially hidden palmette. A wreath of small, paired olive leaves frames the medallion. Three nude women occupy this area. On the left a woman wearing only a necklace and sandals leans against a short pillar while looking at her image in a mirror held in her left hand. A fanciful tendrilled flower grows behind the pillar. The tall central female stands with her left hand braced against her hip and holding a leafy branch in her right hand. She wears a necklace and triangular pendant earring. The third woman is seated on a rock at the right. She wears some drapery gathered across her legs but exposing her torso. Like the central figure, she wears a pendant earring. An Aeolic column stands between these two figures in the background. All three women wear their hair gathered up in a bun. They stand on the exergue, which is decorated with crosshatched triangles.

The engraving is relatively smooth and even. The artist had some difficulty with his drawing of hands and feet. Also, the proportions of the figures, especially their forearms, are very clumsy, and there is little sensitivity in the depiction of hair.

The mirror is typically Praenestine. Its shape may be

compared to No. **39** and especially to a mirror in the Birmingham City Museum, Inv. no. 447.61 (=G. LLOYD-MORGAN in *PBSR* 43 [1975] pl. I). The obverse handle treatment on Nos. **13** and **39** is similar. Parallels for the obverse extension ornament include the Pomerance Praenestine mirror (=*The Pomerance Collection of Ancient Art,* Brooklyn Museum, 1966, no. 126; only the reverse is illustrated). For the subject and style, in addition to the objects mentioned below, compare a Praenestine mirror from Teano: *MonAL* 20 (1910) cols. 79–81, fig. 48.

The engravings on the Detroit mirror have been judged modern by N. DE GRUMMOND, *o.c.,* p. 66. The reason given is an error of "antiquarian detail"; that is, the left female holds a hand mirror with a small cross or hook at the top "unlike any mirrors used in Praeneste or Etruria." It is true that no such mirrors have been recovered to date and that none are depicted in the relatively few shown on other mirrors or engraved cistae. However, such mirrors are illustrated on numerous Etruscan, and especially South Italian, painted vases (e.g., *CVA* Frankfurt 3, Germany 50, pls. 19, 8; 45, 6). Such details, given the well-known stylistic and iconographical influence of South Italian pottery on Praenestine mirrors (see M. CRISTOFANI in *DialArch* 1 [1967] 186–219), could easily crop up in a fourth-century engraving.

In fact, there are at least three cistae (Baltimore 54132; Palestrina 1495 and 1497: BORDENACHE, *Ciste* I, 1, nos. 2, 54, 55) and one mirror (Villa Guilia 51106: A. CIASCA, *Il capitello detto eolico in Etruria,* pl. 24, 1; the drawing in KLÜGMANN-KÖRTE, *ES,* pl. 57, is inaccurate) that, I believe, belong to a single Praenestine workshop, if not the same hand as the Detroit mirror. All show the same peculiar figure style, idiosyncratic details (like the rendering of hair or Aeolic capitals), and even the same vegetal motifs. All were excavated at Palestrina during the nineteenth century, and the authenticity of none has been questioned.

In 1983 I examined the engravings by stereomicroscopy and found that in those portions of engraved lines not having white infilling, the patina was uniformly brown or golden brown. In 1984 G. Carriveau removed the modern infilling and systematically examined the engraved lines with the stereomicroscope. There was no evidence of interruption in the patina. These observations, coupled with the stylistic evidence mentioned above, suggest that both mirror and engravings are ancient.

About 300–275 B.C.

IOWA CITY, IOWA

CLASSICAL MUSEUM
University of Iowa

22. Engraved mirror. Figs. 22a–d.

Inv. 20.73. Provenance: unknown. Purchased in Italy, probably between 1916 and 1925.

R. De Puma in *StEtr* 41 (1973) 159–161, 164–166; fig. la; LI, a–c; R. De Puma in *LIMC* III, *s.v. Dioskouroi, Tinas Cliniar,* no. 42, forthcoming.

Bronze. The mirror was apparently broken into fifteen fragments at some point after acquisition; it is now mended. There are three small lacunae: two roughly triangular areas (1.7 × 0.8 cm.; 0.6 × 0.3 cm.) on the upper disc and a small portion of the lower edge (0.5 × 0.7 cm.). Patina: *Obverse,* bright, powdery green eruptions cover most of the disc. There is considerable flaking and separation of layers along the edge. This continues down the extension and handle, which are encrusted with azurite; the central portion of the handle shows a small patch of smooth brown patina. *Reverse,* a more uniform, dark green incrustation with numerous lighter green eruptions covers the disc. Much separation of layers on the edge and handle.

Measurements: D., 12.2 cm.; Max. H., 23.8 cm.; H. of handle, 11.6 cm.; W. of extension, 2.8 cm.; W. top of handle, 1.5 cm.; W. of terminal, 1.0 cm. Weight, 137.7 cm.

Standard grip mirror with circular disc, concave-sided extension, and handle terminating in a stylized deer's head. Disc and handle cast in one piece. Characteristic section with undecorated edge, small hook on the obverse, and triangular profile on the reverse. There is no central cavity.

Obverse, the unengraved disc is surrounded by the barest vestiges of a beaded border, which once continued to the base of the extension. No trace of ornament remains on the poorly preserved extension. At the top of the handle are four vertical grooves, which may indicate the remains of a floral device, perhaps originally like that on Nos. **2** or **12** (*cf. CSE* Netherlands, nos. 7–8). The handle, whose shaft is now swollen and split by corrosion, was once decorated with short parallel lines along the edge. The deer's head, relatively well preserved, shows the standard features: large

ears firmly pressed against the flat head, bulging eyes, and a large, round muzzle.

Reverse, an olive (or laurel) garland frames the medallion (*cf.* No. **6**). Two youthful males wear chitoniskoi, laced sandals, and piloi; the figure on the right appears to have a himation wrapped about his left arm (*cf.* Biblio. Natl. 1317 = Rebuffat, *Miroir,* pl. 35). These youths lean forward to face each other across a tablelike structure at the center. The "table" is supported by a short pillar topped with an Aeolic capital. The ends of a fillet, apparently tied about the pillar, flutter out from each side of the capital. In a vertical line directly above the capital are a simple lotus bud, a crescent moon, an eight-rayed "star," and a horizontal beam connecting the piloi the two figures wear on their heads. The wavy contour of a rocky groundline frames the medallion. The figures represented are probably the Dioskouroi. For further discussion of the iconography, see R. De Puma, *o.c.,* pp. 164–166.

Compositionally, the mirror belongs to a large group of two-figure arrangements frequently used to depict the twin deities (*cf.* Nos. **1, 8, 34**). Here the figures bend forward to fill the medallion harmoniously. They flank various symbols neatly arranged along a central vertical. The engraving is delicate and of good quality, with no detectable errors or overlappings.

Stylistically, the mirror is related to Gerhard, *ES* I, pl. 48, 2; III, pl. 278, 4; Louvre 1799; Berlin Fr. 96; and no. II la 64 1 in Moscow's State Museum for Pictorial Arts (=A. I. Charsekin, *Zur Deutung etruskischer Sprachdenkmäler,* Frankfurt, 1963, no. 14, p. 78; pl. XI, ill. 15). Biblio. Natl. 1317 (=Rebuffat, *Miroir,* pl. 35; Gerhard, *ES* III, pl. 277, 5) is perhaps the closest stylistic parallel, despite the addition of two figures. See also Sotheby (New York) *Sale Catalogue* 4753Y for 9 December 1981, no. 265.

About 300–250 B.C.

KANSAS CITY, MISSOURI

NELSON-ATKINS MUSEUM OF ART

23. Engraved mirror. Figs. 23a–d.

Inv. 56.124. Provenance: unknown. Given by Katherine Harvey in 1956.

Handbook of the Collections of the Nelson Gallery and Atkins Museum, 4th ed., 1959, p. 31; 5th ed., 1973, p. 42; R. Teitz, *Masterpieces of Etruscan Art* (Worcester, Mass., 1967), pp. 88–89; R. De Puma in *AJA* 88 (1984) 241–242; *LIMC* II (1984) 342, no. 37,c; R. De Puma in *Atti del Secondo Congresso Internazionale Etrusco* (Florence 1986), forthcoming.

Bronze. A deep crack at the top of the extension. The disc is slightly asymmetrical in relation to the handle and the extension. Patina: *Obverse,* good, light green patina over entire surface. This is encrusted with a light oxidation layer which has flaked off in places. There is some surface pitting near the edge and especially at the base of the disc. The handle is still encrusted with dirt. *Reverse,* green patina remains around edge of disc and about 3 cm. into the medallion. Dark green patina in the extension and the handle, which still retains encrusted dirt. The center of the disc appears to have been repolished and is now a dull slate color.

Measurements: Horizontal D., 17 cm.; Vertical D., 16.5 cm.; Max. H., 31.5 cm.; H. of handle, 11.2 cm.; W. of extension, 3.0 cm.; W. top of handle, 2.2 cm.; W. of animal terminal, 1.1 cm. Weight, 476 gr.

Large piriform mirror with broad concave-sided extension and a handle terminating in a vestigial animal head; disc and handle cast in one piece. The flat edge is undecorated. The section is slightly convex and has a shallow hook. The central cavity is about 0.2 cm. in diameter.

Obverse, vestiges of a beaded border surround the disc, extension, and sides of the handle. A shallow groove parallels this border. An engraved palmette with five fronds decorates the extension. Flanking the palmette are two attached volutes and wavy lines, both of which emanate from the palmette's base. Six small circles are symmetrically arranged to each side of the palmette. The handle is modelled with a single large relief area running down its spine (*cf.* No. **21**). The deer-head terminal is modelled only on the top surface. An area of punched dots separates its long ears.

Reverse, the handle is flat and undecorated. The figured scene is framed by a series of paired chevrons, which are probably meant to indicate the paired tips of oblanceolate (laurel?) leaves. This also would explain the paired vertical lines; they must indicate each leaf's rib. These designs move up each side of the disc from the extension's base and meet just to the left of the apex. They are bordered by a pair of parallel lines, which are interrupted only by the crown of the standing male figure on the left. At the center of the extension is a large palmette with seven fronds. An arc of four small circles is symmetrically disposed above it.

Four figures are depicted on the disc. At the right a standing female, wearing a long chiton, sandals, a leafy garland, and an armband of bullae and holding a thyrsos in her right hand, leans forward to embrace a nude young male. The youth wears sandals and a necklace and armband of bullae; he leans backward, arms held awkwardly about the woman's neck, to receive her embrace. To the left of this group stands a tall youthful male holding a leafy staff in his left hand and resting his right hand on his hip. He wears fringed drapery slung about his hips, over his left shoulder and left arm. A fillet is tied about his head and he wears a bulla necklace and sandals. These three figures stand on a series of parallel groundlines. The fourth figure, a small boy, sits on a rock at the left edge of the disc and plays the double flutes. He is nude except for a necklace of three bullae.

This mirror is a replica of a well-known Vulcian example that once belonged to Eduard Gerhard. In 1859 Gerhard's mirror was acquired by the Berlin Museum and is now in the Pergamon Museum in East Berlin. That mirror (no. 3276 = Gerhard, *ES* I, pl. 83) has well-preserved inscriptions that clearly identify the three major figures as Apulu (Apollo), Fufluns (Dionysos), and Semla (Semele). The same subject is certainly intended for the Kansas City mirror, which follows the Berlin model closely. Teitz, *o.c.,* mentions a fragmentary inscription giving the first two letters of Apulu's name above the god's right shoulder. I failed to discern this when examining the object. On the Berlin mirror the flute player has pointed ears and a tail, which characterize him as a youthful satyr. These features have been omitted on the Kansas City mirror.

For the subject and a discussion of the five other mirrors plus additional works in other media with the same representation, see FISCHER-GRAF, pp. 64–72; PFISTER-ROESGEN, *Spiegel,* pp. 76–81; and G. BATTAGLIA in *Rend-Linc* 7 (1930) 275–290. Although the mirrors themselves are ancient, the engravings on all of them appear to be modern. In some cases the style is extremely clumsy and inept (Biblio. Natl. 1303 = REBUFFAT, *Miroir,* pp. 411–412; pl. 83). On one mirror the engraving was executed on the reflecting obverse instead of the normal reverse side (Biblio. Natl. 1301 = REBUFFAT, *Miroir,* pp. 409–411; pl. 83). See also I. KRAUSKOPF in *LIMC* II (1984) 342, nos. 36–37.

Often, various details of the Berlin mirror have been omitted or changed by the modern copyists who probably worked from the published engravings of the original, which appeared as early as 1833 (*cf. MonIst* 1 [1829–1833] pl. 56, 2). The following variants occur on the Kansas City mirror: the satyr's tail and pointed ears are omitted from the small flutist; his right foot is missing; the top of his left foot seems to have been misunderstood as the lower hem of Apollo's drapery; the fingers of his left hand are missing; the rock on which he sits is given added interior detail. Apollo wears simpler sandals; his necklace contains an additional bulla; the way in which his hair winds over and behind his fillet (*cf.* the bronze Apollo from the House of the Citharist, Pompeii) is completely misunderstood; and the drapery that should fall behind his left arm is missing. Dionysos wears oddly drawn sandals (he is barefoot in the original and all other copies) and his left foot is positioned differently; his hair does not fall behind his left arm and reappear below it. Semele, like Apollo, wears very simplified sandals and her left foot does not point outward but is shown in profile; her drapery is perfunctorily executed; the wreath she wears is much less complicated; and the base of her thyrsos has been omitted. The border is completely different from the Berlin original and cannot be paralleled by any mirror known to me.

Results of stereomicroscopic examination of the patina and the engravings are also relevant here. The engraved extension ornament on the obverse is deep, firm, and confident; corrosion products within the lines and beside them are identical. The engravings on the reverse are shallow, thin, even sketchy. They often penetrate layers of corrosion.

My conclusions, based on style as well as the physical examination of engravings and patina, are that the mirror and the engravings on the obverse are ancient. It should be noted that the distinctive piriform shape is characteristic of mirrors made at Praeneste (*cf.* Nos. **13, 14, 20, 21, 38, 39**) and that many unengraved mirrors (i.e., undecorated on the reverse) have been found (*cf.* No. **38** and a close parallel from TEANO in *MonAL* 20 [1910] col. 108, fig. 78). The engravings on the reverse are modern, probably inspired by and copied from the 1833 engraving of the mirror now in East Berlin. The modern engravings are closest in style to those on the replica now in Syracuse.

Praenestine mirror, *ca.* 300 B.C., with modern engravings on the reverse.

LAWRENCE, KANSAS

WILCOX COLLECTION
University of Kansas Classics Department

24. Engraved mirror. Figs. 24a–d.

No Inv. Provenance: unknown. Purchased from George Allen (Philadelphia dealer) in 1968.

Hesperia Art, *Bulletin* 43 (1968), item A 18; *Handbook of the Collection: Helen Foresman Spencer Museum of Art* (Lawrence 1978), ill. on p. 13.

Bronze. Intact and in fair condition. Patina: *Obverse,* very heavy incrustations of dark green and light green carbonates. A small patch of smooth, dark green-brown bronze appears at the lower left of disc. Areas of dirt obscure the handle decoration. *Reverse,* dark green areas on handle and edge of disc. Medallion has small patches of light green eruptions, but the background is mostly yellow with scattered patches of dark red.

Measurements: D., 11.9 cm.; Max. H., 23.6 cm.; H. of handle, 8.8 cm.; W. of extension, 2.5 cm.; W. top of handle, 1.8 cm.; W. of terminal, 1.0 cm. Weight, 154.9 gr.

Standard grip mirror with circular disc, concave-sided extension, and handle terminating in a stylized deer's head. Disc and handle cast in one piece. The section shows a gentle convexity and a pair of parallel grooves at edge of obverse; on the reverse the medallion border is very slightly raised above the medallion. The central cavity is 0.1 cm. in diameter.

Obverse, the unengraved disc is surrounded by a pair of parallel grooves; the edge is marked by a series of deep radiating notches (*cf.* Nos. **1, 8, 28, 34, 36**). The extension contains a typical flame motif (*cf.* Nos. **1, 5, 6, 8, 10, 27, 28, 33, 34, 36**). The central stem of the handle shows vestiges of two opposed animal heads. The terminal, in the shape of a deer's head, is obscured by heavy corrosion.

Reverse, a spiky garland frames the medallion (*cf.* Nos. **3, 28, 36**). In this case the garland consists of overlapping

trifoliate leaves, which are longer and sharper than usual (*cf.* Nos. **3, 28**). "Slide binders" appear at top and bottom but not sides. A floral device, consisting of three pointed leaves apparently bound at midpoint, decorates the extension. A series of irregular punched dots appears below this on the handle.

The medallion shows a typical four-figure composition. Two identical males, each wearing Phrygian caps, knee-length tunics, and cross-strapped sandals, lean against short Ionic piers on either side of the medallion. An idiosyncratic detail of this engraver is his use of short arcs that rise upward from the hems of the tunics. Between these males are two women facing them. The one on the left wears a Phrygian cap and long chiton; her right arm appears to embrace the back of the male on her right (*cf.* Nos. **5, 27, 33**). The other female is nude except for high-laced boots and some drapery, which is tucked between her thighs and appears also to be draped about her right shoulder and arm. For a similar treatment, see B. Laubie in *Revue Archéologique de l'Est et du Centre-Est* 14 (1963) 293–297, especially fig. 84. Several small arcs help to emphasize details of her anatomy. Her hair is rendered by a series of overlapping circular forms. For discussion of the subject, see Nos. **5, 6,** and **27** and the variants, Nos. **33** and **36.**

The composition is among the most popular on Etruscan mirrors: two symmetrical figures flank two more contrasted figures who turn outward to engage them in conversation. The engraving is firm and consistent. There are numerous overlappings and some awkward omissions. For two related mirrors, see Gerhard, *ES* III, pl. 277, 3, and Klügmann-Körte, *ES,* pl. 84, 1. The obverse treatment is paralleled by mirrors in Bologna (=*CSE* Bologna I, no. 5) and Leiden (*CSE* Netherlands, nos. 12, 19).

Late third century B.C.

MILWAUKEE, WISCONSIN

MILWAUKEE PUBLIC MUSEUM

25. Engraved mirror. Figs. 25a–d.

Inv. N11610. Provenance: unknown. Purchased from Münzen und Medaillen (Basel) in 1963.

Kunstwerke der Antike, Auktion XXVI (5 October 1963), p. 18, no. 35; pl. 10; R. De Puma in *Muse, Annual of the Museum of Art and Archaeology* 20 (1986), forthcoming.

Bronze. Several large cracks at the edge near bottom of disc. There is a small triangular lacuna at lower right (reverse) of disc. Portions of this area on the obverse have been restored. Patina: *Obverse,* green and dark brown cover most of the disc's surface. Near the center are areas of bright green and red-orange incrustations. Some very small patches of shiny bronze appear above the extension. The tang is green and dark brown with a fair amount of pitting. *Reverse,* dark, even, brown and green patina over most of the disc. Areas of powdery, light green corrosion near the edge. Some areas of roughness, pitting, and scratching, especially on left and base of disc. The central cavity is shallow, semicircular in profile, and 0.2 cm. in diameter.

Measurements: D., 15.1 cm.; Max. H., 19.7 cm.; L. of tang, 2.6 cm.; W. of extension, 2.7 cm. Weight, 115.4 gr.

Circular mirror with small extension and a rounded tang. The edge is undecorated. The section shows a very thin disc and a slight concavity on the reverse with the edge profile rising to a sharp point (*cf. CSE* Netherlands, nos. 3, 29; *CSE* Denmark 1, nos. 16, 23).

Obverse, vestiges of an engraved volute decorate the extension. At the top of the extension are two juxtaposed volutes whose outer ends are no longer visible. A few faint traces of vertical lines between them suggest that a radiating palmette composed of five fronds once ornamented this area. For a similar design, see *CSE* Denmark 1, figs. 16c–d.

Reverse, a large nude warrior charges to the left. He wears an Attic helmet with neck-guard and high frontlet terminating in a volute above his ear. (This type of helmet is discussed by A. Snodgrass, *Arms and Armour of the Greeks* [Ithaca 1967], pp. 69; 138, n. 29; *cf.* Gerhard, *ES* II, pl. 230 = Thorvaldsens Museum H 2168.) The warrior also wears a himation, which falls from his shoulders, and one shoe on his left foot. He brandishes a battle ax in his right hand and holds a large, undecorated shield on his left arm. The warrior's head is in profile and resembles the head of the Lasa on No. **18.** Anatomical details are simple but powerful. The outer line of the right thigh and knee is missing (*cf. CSE* Denmark 1, no. 5). A large stylized flower appears at the left edge of the disc.

This mirror is clearly related in style and type to a large series of tang mirrors depicting a single running or flying figure with large, stylized plants often shown in the field. A number of mirrors of this same type show a winged Minerva wearing the same kind of Attic helmet and carrying the same large shield (e.g., Gerhard, *ES* I, pl. 36, 7). A larger group of parallels, some from datable contexts, depict Lasae (*cf.* Nos. **2, 18**). The best parallels come from Tarquinian tombs and date between *ca.* 300 and 250 B.C. An exact parallel with an armed warrior has not been located. For a similar figure, compare the satyr on a mirror from Arezzo (Klügmann-Körte, *ES,* p. 50, no. 40a).

In composition and style the Milwaukee mirror is closely related to No. **18.** Here the large flower and shield replace the Lasa's unfurled wings as framing elements for the warrior whose pose is almost identical.

300–250 B.C.

MINNEAPOLIS, MINNESOTA

MINNEAPOLIS INSTITUTE OF ARTS

26. Engraved mirror. Figs. 26a-d.

Inv. 57.14 (formerly 57.198). Provenance: near Orvieto. Formerly in the Elie Borowski Collection. Given by Mrs. Lyndon M. King in 1957.

KLÜGMANN-KÖRTE, *ES,* p. 209; pl. 158; P. JACOBSTHAL, *Der Blitz in der orientalischen und griechischen Kunst* (Berlin 1906) p. 12; DUCATI, *RM* 1912, p. 246, fig. 1; MATTHIES, *PS,* p. 10; DU-CATI, *AE* I, p. 330; C. KOCH, *Gestirnverehrung im alten Italien* (Frankfurt 1933), p. 57; MANSUELLI, *StEtr 1943,* pp. 497–498; MANSUELLI, *StEtr 1946–47,* pp. 14; 49, no. 4; BEAZLEY, *JHS 1949,* p. 2, fig. 1; O. W. VON VACANO, *Die Etrusker* (Stuttgart 1955), p. 179, fig. 77; MAYER-PROKOP, *Griffspiegel,* pp. 12–13, 46–47; pl. 3, 2; D. G. MITTEN and S. DOERINGER, *Master Bronzes from the Classical World* (Mainz 1967), p. 210, no. 214; P. E. ARIAS in *StEtr* 37 (1969) 32, fig. 2; PFIFFIG, *Religio,* pp. 241–242, fig. 105; J. P. OLESON in *AJA* 79 (1975) 195; pl. 37, fig. 7; H. JUCKER in G. Kopcke and M. Moore, eds., *Studies in Classical Art and Archaeology: A Tribute to P. H. von Blanckenhagen* (Locust Valley, N.J., 1979) p. 55, n. 12; p. 61, n. 54; R. DE PUMA in *RM* 87 (1980) 26, fig. 9A (disc section); M. TIRELLI in *StEtr* 49 (1981) 42, no. 3; pl. XV, c; DE GRUMMOND, *Guide,* p. 142; fig. 81.

Bronze. Intact but heavily pitted, especially on the obverse. The disc is slightly warped and thinner than the tang. Patina: *Obverse,* dark brown patina with even pitting over most of the disc; the tang is better preserved. There is an irregular patch of shinier bronze at center of disc. Some tiny surface cracks. *Reverse,* very dark brown over most surfaces but smooth and shiny on extension and upper left disc. The center of disc may have been polished in recent times. Tang and right side of disc are heavily pitted.

Measurements: D., 13.3 cm.; Max. H., 19.8 cm.; H. of tang, 5.3 cm.; W. of extension, 3.0 cm.; Max. W. of tang, 1.0 cm. Weight, 226.6 gr.

Circular mirror with long tang and curved extension. The section is flat and of uniform thickness. The central cavity (just to the left of the engraved figure's earlobe) is circular, 0.1 cm. in diameter, and has vertical sides.

Obverse, all decoration is confined to the extension and disc area immediately above it. A pair of engraved symmetrical volutes fits snugly into the contours of the extension. A

pair of small palmette leaves springs upward from their point of contact; a single leaf points down, on axis with the tang. Another smaller pair of volutes and two tendrils, terminating in ivy leaves, complete the design on the disc.

Reverse, a pair of volutes, inverted versions of those on the obverse, ornaments the extension. Two horizontal lines are engraved on the long tang. A wave-crest pattern borders the disc. It flows in opposite directions from the extension and meets at the top of the disc. In addition, a pair of converging lines rising from the volutes of the extension carries four more wave crests on each side. There is some confusion as to how these should relate to the wave-crest border. Forming an exergue above this is a third area of wave crests.

The arms and upper torso of a youthful nude male appear above the exergue. His chest and outstretched arms are shown frontally; his head is in left profile. His long hair consists of a series of hooklike curls which emerge from a fillet. He holds two curious objects in his upturned hands. These objects are indicated by circles (the one on the left is smaller and held lower than that on the right) from which three wavy lines radiate upward. Above or behind the figure's head is a large crescent from which nine rays emanate.

Most commentators have identified this figure as the sun god Helios-Usil rising from the sea. Judging from the upward direction of the radiating glow of the fiery globes the god holds, OLESON, *o.c.,* probably is correct in suggesting a setting sun. Although other representations of the sun god exist in Etruscan art (see TIRELLI, *o.c.*), this mirror is a unique depiction of the setting (or rising) sun. See also the figure (Cautha ?) on a gold ring from Aléria dating *ca.* 325–300 B.C. (E. SIMON in M. Cristofani et al., *Gli Etruschi, una nuova immagine* [Florence 1984], p. 156).

For two mirrors with somewhat related scenes and ornamental borders, see MAYER-PROKOP, *Griffspiegel,* pl. 48, 1–2. The style of Usil's profile and curls is also reminiscent of the running athletes on the right wall of the Tomba delle Olimpiadi and the reclining banqueter on the right wall or the youthful dancer on the back wall of the Tomba delle Lionesse, both at Tarquinia. Similar radiant haloes appear on other mirrors with Usil depictions: MAYER-PROKOP, *Griffspiegel,* pls. 2–3; TIRELLI, *o.c.;* PFISTER-ROESGEN, *Spiegel,* pp. 107–109.

The symmetrical composition and the use of an exergue are typical of archaic mirror designs. The engravings are deep, strong, and consistent on the reverse; the obverse engravings are relatively lighter and weaker. The only noticeable error on the reverse is the double engraving of the figure's right elbow.

500–460 B.C.

27. Engraved mirror. Figs. 27a–d.

Inv. 62.13. Provenance: unknown. Given by Robert E. Hecht, Jr., in 1962.

R. DE PUMA in *StEtr* 41 (1973) 163, 170; fig. 1, d; pl. LIV, a–c.

Bronze. Intact and in good condition. Patina: *Obverse,* bright green and dark blue corrosion covers most of the upper half of disc. The lower half is still encrusted with dirt. The extension has the smoothest and hardest patina, while the handle is powdery. Small wax deposits appear at center of disc and on the terminal. *Reverse,* light, powdery green incrustations over a matt, dark brown background with some isolated patches of dark blue cuprite. Several small areas of encrusted dirt, especially on the rim.

Measurements: D., 13.2. cm.; Max. H., 26.4 cm.; H. of handle, 10.3 cm.; W. of extension, 3.3 cm.; W. top of handle, 2.1 cm.; W. of terminal, 1.3 cm. Weight, 256.4 gr.

Standard grip mirror with circular disc, concave-sided extension, and handle terminating in a deer's head. Disc and handle cast in one piece. The section shows the characteristic hook and triangle profile at the edge, a pronounced shelf for the medallion's border ornament, and the usual concavity of the reverse. The central cavity is perfectly round and 0.1 cm. in diameter.

Obverse, a deep groove surrounds the disc and continues to the ends of the extension. Paralleling this on the outside is a crudely executed beaded border. The extension shows a classic example of the flame motif (*cf.* Nos. **1, 5, 6**). Here the leaves are carefully striated. The handle is decorated with juxtaposed griffin heads and terminates in a stylized deer's head.

Reverse, a tightly wrought cable pattern borders the medallion. The extension shows vestiges of what most likely was once an engraved lotus bud (*cf.* Nos. **5, 22**). Corrosion obscures any decoration on the handle.

The medallion shows a typical four-figure composition (*cf.* Nos. **5, 6, 24, 33, 36**). Two males lean against small pillars on either side of the disc and face inward. They wear piloi and elaborately rendered tunics. The tunics have large, billowy tops with belts (?) at the waist, unusual cross designs on the skirts, and an odd flap or fold (indicated by short parallel diagonals) on the side. These folds are surely abstractions indicating that the innermost arm of each figure is wrapped in a himation (*cf.* GERHARD, *ES* I, pl. 47, 2–4).

The male figures flank two females, one clothed, one nude. The clothed female raises her right arm to touch the male to her right (*cf.* No. **5**, where the same gesture occurs). She wears a long chiton, whose top resembles those of the men, and a strange, pointed hat. The nude female stands in the typical hipshot pose with right hand behind her hip and some drapery tucked between her thighs. Her head is shown in three-quarter view looking toward the male to her left. She wears a kestos (*cf.* No. **28**, where it is worn by Hera-Uni; for other examples, see GERHARD, *ES* III, pl. 278, 3, 5, 6). A crudely drawn pediment appears behind and above the figures' heads; there also are indications of a rocky groundline at the sides of the medallion.

Subject: the Dioskouroi with Minerva and Aphrodite (or Helen?). See discussion of No. **5**. The kestos is normally associated with the goddess Aphrodite-Turan but may be worn by others.

The design and composition are standard. Although idiosyncratic, the engraving is consistent and strong. There are several overlappings, especially in the rendering of drapery folds.

Late second century B.C.

OBERLIN, OHIO

ALLEN MEMORIAL ART MUSEUM
Oberlin College

28. Engraved mirror. Figs. 28a–d.

Inv. 42.122. Provenance: near Tarquinia. In 1878 the mirror was in the collection of Pasinati, a Roman antiquities dealer. Later it appears to have been in the collection of Louis E. Lord. It was in Oberlin before 1937 but unaccessioned until 1942. It was purchased (apparently from Lord) through the R. T. Miller, Jr. Fund.

CII, App., p. 66, no. 772; Klügmann-Körte, *ES,* pp. 126–127; pl. 98, 2; L. Lord in *AJA* 41 (1937) 602–606; figs. 5, 7; R. Bloch in *MEFR* 62 (1950) 94–98; fig. 22; C. Picard in *RA* 37 (1951) 218; C. Clairmont, *Das Parisurteil in der Antiken Kunst,* Zurich 1951, p. 67, K207; *Allen Memorial Art Museum Bulletin* 11, 2 (1954) ill. at no. 7; 16, 2 (1959) p. 119; 16, 3 (1959) ill. on p. 168; D. G. Mitten and S. F. Doeringer, *Master Bronzes from the Classical World,* Mainz 1967, no. 218, p. 215; Rebuffat, *Miroir,* pp. 466–467; pl. 86; L. Bonfante in *GettyMusJ* 8 (1980) 152, fig. 8; J. Petit in *RLouvre* 31, 1 (1981) 30–31, fig. 5; *LIMC* II (1984) 172, no. 19. Inscriptions: De Simone I, p. 57 (11); *Thes. L.E. I,* pp. 125, 240, 349, 357.

Bronze. Large sections of the lower disc's rim are missing. A major crack runs across disc from center right (reverse) to lower left. There is a tiny hole in the gouged area at lower left. A small perforation occurs on the upper right portion of the extension paralleling the border. The lower left disc is heavily gouged; engravings in this area are lost. Several damaged patches on the obverse have been filled in. The lower disc is considerably warped. Patina: *Obverse,* much of the disc is shiny bronze with tiny surface cracks, especially at center, and several scratches caused by careless cleaning. There are a number of large patches of green incrustation about the perimeter of disc and especially in grooves. The extension has areas of light green incrustation but is generally clean. The handle has a light green corrosion within recessed grooves and decoration. Higher areas are shiny bronze, the result of handling. *Reverse,* most of the disc is covered by a dark brown or matt green patina. Shiny bronze patches occur at extreme edge of the disc. Some patches of white corrosion appear in damaged areas at right edge. There are very fine cracks near center of disc and light green, powdery incrustations on extension and in recesses of the handle. Otherwise, both areas are an even dark green or matt brown except for high projections of shiny bronze.

Measurements: D., 12.4 cm.; Max. H., 24.6 cm.; L. of handle, 9.0 cm.; W. of extension, 3.5 cm.; W. of terminal, 1.6 cm. Weight, 338 gr.

Circular mirror with concave-sided extension and elaborately modelled, massive handle. Disc and handle cast in one piece. The disc section shows the raised medallion border and heavy rim profile with a single groove on the obverse typical of the "Kranzspiegelgruppe" (*cf.* Nos. **3, 24, 36;** *CSE* Netherlands, no. 12). The thick edge (0.7 cm.) is decorated with a series of deep notches (*cf.* especially No. **24**). The central cavity is circular and 0.16 cm. in diameter.

Obverse, the expansion of the edge's deep notches is checked by a small channel running around the disc and terminating at the extension's points. A row of small punched circles abuts the channel and follows its entire length (*cf.* Rebuffat, *Miroir,* pl. 9 = Biblio. Natl. 1291). The extension is decorated with two broad but shallow grooves, which gradually touch at the extension's narrowest point. Here their tips are rounded and flare out to accommodate a flamelike element (*cf.* Nos. **1, 5, 6, 8, 10, 24, 27, 33, 34, 36**). Below is a pointed leaf covered with rows of tiny punched dots.

The handle is particularly well preserved. It terminates in a large ram's head. Above, at the midpoint of the handle, are two juxtaposed griffin heads. Higher still, reaching to the base of the extension, are two elegant acanthus leaves which spread their tips to meet the extension's points. All of this area is enlivened by rich modelling and punch marks. See No. **3** for a similar treatment; *cf.* Rebuffat, *Miroir,* pl. 1 (= Biblio. Natl. 1283).

Reverse, the modelled underside of the ram's head is covered with short engraved arcs to indicate the striations of wool. The central portion of the handle above the terminal is filled with rows of large punch marks. The extension is engraved with an elaborate lotus bud device springing from a volute base (*cf.* Gerhard, *ES* IV, pl. 385 = British Museum 714; Lambrechts, *Mir. Mus. Royaux,* no. 1 = Brussels R 1251 bis; *CSE* Netherlands, no. 12). The area at the base of this design is covered with small punch marks neatly confined beneath two arcs.

A plain, offset band (*ca.* 1.2 cm. wide) encloses the disc and extension. Four labels, one near each of the figures in the medallion, are inscribed retrograde on the upper part of this band. Each name is bracketed by a double interpoint. From left to right they read:

elaxśntre

turan

uni

[m]e̜nrfa

Very few of the many mirrors depicting the Judgment of Paris have all the characters identified by inscription (*cf.* I. JUCKER in *MusHelv* 39 [1982] 5–14 for an earlier example).

The figure of Alexandros (Elexsntre or Elexsantre) sits on a rocky shelf at the extreme left of the medallion. He wears a Phrygian cap, a himation wrapped about his thighs, and high-laced boots. A strap, perhaps belonging to a scabbard, crosses his chest from the right shoulder. His left hand holds a gnarled club which rests against his right leg. A small tree grows between Alexandros and Aphrodite (Turan), the next figure. She is nude except for high-laced boots, a bracelet on her left wrist, and a diadem. She stands with left hand on hip in an elegant three-quarter back view as she gazes at Alexandros.

The tallest figure, that of Hera (Uni), stands at the disc's center. She wears the same high-laced boots, bracelets on each wrist, a torque (incorrectly drawn in KLÜGMANN-KÖRTE, *ES,* pl. 98, 2), and a fringed kestos. A piece of drapery hangs from her left shoulder and is wrapped about her right leg. She looks to the right in the direction of the fourth figure, Minerva (Menrfa), separated from her by a second small tree. The third goddess wears a short-sleeved chiton, a scaly aegis, helmet, and bracelet. She holds a spear in her left hand; her shield is propped against the right edge of the medallion. Few anatomical details appear on the females; those on the body of Alexandros are indicated with short, irregular clusters of concentric semicircles and arcs. The entire scene is framed by a spiky garland with four so-called slide binders indicated at the cardinal points (*cf.* No. 3).

For discussion of this theme, see LORD, *o.c.;* CLAIRMONT, *o.c.,* especially pp. 65–76, for representations on mirrors; I. JUCKER in *MusHelv* 39 (1982) 5–14.

REBUFFAT, *Miroir,* pp. 466–467, has correctly associated the Oberlin mirror with three others that almost certainly came from the same workshop, "graveurs du groupe de l'Oberlin College." These mirrors are (1) from Bolsena (=BLOCH, *o.c.,* p. 93, fig. 21); (2) from Vulci (=Villa Giulia 63364: U. FERRAGUTI in *StEtr* 11 [1937] 110, fig. 3; M. T. FALCONI AMORELLI in *ArchCl* 28 [1976] 236; pl. 86, b, image reversed; pl. 89, b); and (3) Dresden ZV 30,2 (=*CSE* DDR 2, no. 6, forthcoming). To this we may add (4) Paris, Petit Palais, no. DUT 1616 (=*RLouvre* 31, 1 [1982] 27–34), which is similar to example 1, and (5) a mirror formerly in the Museo Penacchi at Perugia (=GERHARD, *ES* III, pl. 263, 5). This last example is particularly close to example 1 and is probably the mirror now in the St. Louis Art Museum (our No. **36**).

The similarities among all six examples are striking, although a seated male substitutes for Minerva and a temple façade replaces the two trees on the Oberlin mirror. The positions of the two nude goddesses are virtually repeated, although Hera's left arm is now bent at the elbow. Each version of this figure wears the distinctive torque, fringed kestos, and drapery tucked between her legs (*cf.* KLÜGMANN-KÖRTE, *ES,* pls. 88, 2; 102, 2; and GERHARD, *ES* III, pl. 257C). The figure corresponding to Alexandros has also moved his left arm in the five related mirrors. Stylistically and typologically, the mirror is also closely related to KLÜGMANN-KÖRTE, *ES,* pl. 118; note especially the similarity of female hairstyles.

About 300 B.C.

OMAHA, NEBRASKA

JOSLYN ART MUSEUM

29. Unengraved mirror. Fig. 29a.

Inv. 1934.268. Provenance: unknown. Given to the museum by Mrs. C. N. Dietz in 1934.

Unpublished.

Bronze. Intact and in good condition. Patina: *Obverse,* smooth, matt brown surface interrupted by areas of light green eruptions. *Reverse,* similar to obverse but with two areas of white and light green incrustations. A small patch of modern shellac or glue on upper left edge.

Measurements: D., 14.9 cm.; Max. H., 16.0 cm.; L. of tang, 2.1 cm.; Max. W. of tang, 1.5 cm. Weight, 294 gr.

Mirror with elliptical disc and short tang cast in one piece. The disc section shows the perfectly flat profile (*cf.* Nos. **26, 32**) frequent on early mirrors. There is no central cavity. There is no engraved or modelled decoration.

Parallels for this mirror include *CSE* Bologna II, no. 24 (*cf.* nos. 16 and 23 as well); Beazley-Magi, pl. 53, no. 18; Lambrechts, *Mir. Mus. Royaux,* no. 62 (=Brussels R 1311). Also compare Comstock-Vermeule, *Boston Bronzes,* no. 392.

Probably 500–450 B.C.

30. Unengraved mirror. Fig. 30a.

Inv. 1936.377. Provenance: unknown. Given to the museum by Mrs. A. F. Jonas in 1936.

Unpublished.

Bronze. Intact except for a small hole in the center of the disc. The center is dented from the obverse. Patina: *Obverse,* dark green with generalized areas of cuprite and white incrustations. *Reverse,* brown or bright green with an even distribution of brown or green eruptions.

Measurements: D., 13.2 cm.; Max. H., 16.4 cm.; L. of tang, 3.1 cm.; Max. W. of tang, 0.9 cm. Weight, 133 gr.

Mirror with circular disc and small tang with a rounded end cast in one piece. The disc section is flat. No evidence of a central cavity remains. There is no engraved or modelled decoration. This mirror's shape and size are close to two others: *CSE* Bologna II, nos. 7 and 18.

Probably 475–425 B.C.

31. Mirror handle. Figs. 31a–b.

Inv. 1936.359. Provenance: unknown. Given to the museum by Mrs. A. F. Jonas in 1936.

Unpublished.

Bronze. Intact and in excellent condition. Patina: smooth, even, dark green patina on all sides.

Measurements: Max. H., 10.1 cm.; Max. W., 4.5 cm.; W. of terminal, 0.9 cm. Weight, 42 gr.

Solid cast mirror handle with deer-head terminal familiar from numerous examples. The handle above the terminal consists of a polygonal shaft with two bulging areas decorated with beading and separated from the shaft by relief bands. At the top end of the shaft is an elliptical area from which springs the attachment. This is in the form of three deeply modelled leaves.

There are several parallels of various sizes for this handle. One example of precisely the same dimensions and almost identical design is Bryn Mawr College M–75 (=K. M. Phillips in *StEtr* 36 [1968] pl. 25, a–b). Other parallels include Gerhard, *ES* I, pl. 60, 1 and 4; Lambrechts, *Mir. Mus. Royaux,* nos. 56 and 57; *CSE* Denmark 1, nos. 17 and 18; *CSE* Netherlands, nos. 16 and 27; *CSE* Bologna I, no. 22; S. Boucher, *Bronzes grecs, hellénistiques et étrusques des Musées de Lyon* (Lyon 1970) 129, no. 136. A Praenestine example of comparable size and design comes from a datable context, *ca.* 250–200 B.C. See G. Battaglia in *NS* 11 (1933) 184–185, fig. 4.

Third century B.C.

ROCKFORD, ILLINOIS

Rockford College Art Collection

32. Unengraved mirror. Figs. 32a–b.

Inv. 7. Provenance: unknown. Purchased by Frank and Fannie Jewett from Aziz Khayat (New York dealer) in the 1920s.

Unpublished.

Bronze. Intact and in fair condition. There is one large crack to the left of the tang on the obverse; the tang itself is also cracked. A Roman bronze Silenos or Bacchus head in left profile was attached to the Etruscan disc sometime before acquisition. Patina: both sides are heavily corroded with dark green incrustations. There are a few patches of powdery, light green eruptions on the disc. The central portion of the tang is purple and dark brown on the obverse.

Measurements: D., 12.0 cm.; Max. H., 16.9 cm.; L. of tang, 5.4 cm.; Max. W. of tang, 1.1 cm.

Circular mirror with long, flat tang. The section reveals the thick, flat profile characteristic of early mirrors. There is no central cavity now visible. The mirror is unengraved. Parallels for the shape include *CSE* Bologna I, no. 27, and II, no. 17, both assigned to the fifth century B.C.

Probably 450–425 B.C.

33. Engraved mirror. Figs. 33a–d.

Inv. 124. Provenance: unknown. Purchased by Frank and Fannie Jewett from Aziz Khayat (New York dealer) in the 1920s.

Unpublished.

Bronze. Intact and in good condition. Two minor cracks along the edge of the disc. Patina: *Obverse,* very dark brown patina uniformly covering the disc and handle. There is considerable flaking and some pitting on the disc. *Reverse,* dark brown, almost black, patina over disc and handle. There are numerous patches of a dark purple incrustation on the disc.

Measurements: D., 12.9 cm.; Max. H., 26.3 cm.; H. of handle, 9.9 cm.; W. of extension, 2.7 cm.; W. top of handle, 0.7 cm.; W. of terminal, 1.2 cm. Weight, 232 gr.

Standard grip mirror with circular disc, concave-sided extension, and deer-head handle terminal. Disc and handle cast in one piece. The section has the standard features of this type of mirror (see Nos. **5, 6, 8**). The central cavity is round in section and 0.1 cm. in diameter.

Obverse, a deep groove surrounds the disc and continues down the sides of the extension. A standard flame motif decorates the extension (*cf.* Nos. **1, 5, 6, 8, 24, 27, 28, 34, 36**). Juxtaposed griffin heads and a terminal in the shape of a deer's head form the handle. The top of the deer's head is marked by small, wavy engravings to indicate the striations of the animal's skin.

Reverse, a simple cable pattern, ineptly formed at the base, frames the medallion. A typical lotus bud ornaments the extension (*cf.* Nos. **2, 5, 22, 24, 28**). A row of punch marks runs down the handle but is replaced by three short rows of curved gouges on the underside of the terminal.

The medallion shows four figures. Two males, virtually mirror-images of each other, stand on the sides and face the center. They wear Phrygian caps, long sleeveless tunics belted above the waist, and high, laced sandals. The one on the left also appears to have some drapery wrapped about his left arm. Both figures lean on perfunctorily drawn Ionic pedestals. Two figures stand between these males. On the left a female, who wears a Phrygian cap and a long chiton, faces left and extends her right arm toward the male. The gesture seems to indicate that her hand would be placed on his right shoulder, but it is not visible. Standing beside her, but turned toward the right, is a nude male with long hair wearing only laced sandals. He stands in a familiar pose repeated on numerous other mirrors of this type (*cf.* Nos. **5, 6, 24**).

Two other features complete the picture: a series of

four horizontal lines stretch behind the heads of the figures but are omitted at the center; a wavy line moves behind the male at the right edge of the medallion. The first lines are no doubt the vestiges of an architectural background, usually a pediment, frequently depicted on mirrors. The wavy lines often indicate framing groundlines or clouds.

This mirror represents a common variant of the standard four-figure composition. See discussion for No. **5**. Here the nude female is replaced by a nude male, although the same pose is maintained by all four figures. On mirrors of this general type with inscriptions, the nude male is identified as Menelaus (Menle), Polydeukes (Pultuce), Ajax (Efas), and Agamemnon (Achmem...), to name a few. Again, we see that the four-figure mirrors do not represent a standard scene from mythology; they can become whatever is required by the simple addition of inscriptions.

The design and composition are simple and represent a variant of the more common type where two males flank two females. The engraving is shallow and irregular, especially in the rendering of drapery. There are several overlappings and omissions, especially the right contour of the nude male (*cf.* No. **24** and a mirror on the London market in *Architectural Digest* 40, 6 [June 1983] 145) and the horizontal lines of the architectural setting.

Sylistic parallels for this mirror include GERHARD, *ES* III, pl. 266, 2 (=Louvre 1784); pls. 266, 1; 266, 5; REBUFFAT, *Miroir*, pls. 23, 36, 69, and 70; E. WILLIAMS, *The Archaeological Collection of the Johns Hopkins University* (Baltimore 1984) no. 51, pp. 73–76.

200–150 B.C.

34. Engraved mirror. Figs. 34a–d.

Inv. 125. Provenance: unknown. Purchased by Frank and Fannie Jewett from Aziz Khayat (New York dealer) in the 1920s.

Unpublished. R. DE PUMA in *RM* 87 (1980) 26, fig. 9F (disc section).

Bronze. There are several large cracks on the disc. A small lacuna (0.3 × 0.5 cm.) occurs at the heel of the left figure. Patina: *Obverse*, a good, blue and light green patina covers the entire object. There are numerous scratches and some encrusted dirt on the disc. The handle has a fine, uniform, and smooth, light green patina. *Reverse*, similar to obverse but with more encrusted dirt and several patches of a darker green patina, especially on the extension and handle.

Measurements: D., 11.7 cm.; Max. H., 23.7 cm.; H. of handle, 9.3 cm.; W. of extension, 2.6 cm.; W. top of handle, 1.9 cm.; W. of terminal, 1.0 cm. Weight, 129 gr.

Standard grip mirror with circular disc, concave-sided extension, and deer-head handle terminal. Disc and handle cast in one piece. The section has a sharp, flat edge and pronounced concavity (*cf.* REBUFFAT, *Miroir*, pl. 106, no. 1311). The central cavity is 0.1 cm. in diameter.

Obverse, a series of radiating notches or dentils backed by a single engraved line forms the border around disc and extension. A flame motif decorates the extension (see No. **33**). Rows of small, square punch marks embellish this motif. Cursory markings on the handle indicate that a simplified version of the juxtaposed griffin-head motif (*cf.* No. **28**) was attempted. The deer-head terminal is clearly defined by engraved striations and lines for its features.

Reverse, there is a raised border, but it is undecorated. The extension simply shows paired curves echoing the concave sides. The handle is undecorated. The medallion shows two highly stylized male figures, who stand facing each other with outer arms bent, hands on hips, and one leg crossed behind the other. Each wears a Phrygian cap and a sleeveless tunic, which is belted or gathered across the chest and reaches to the knees. Between the figures are two pairs of horizontal lines, probably indicating the dokana (see No. **22**). Behind the figures appear stylized, conical shields.

This is a simple, straightforward composition based on more complex and presumably earlier designs showing the Dioskouroi (*cf.* Nos. **1, 8, 22**). Engravings are shallow but fluid and controlled. There are overlappings (e.g., in the upper portions of the tunics) and omissions (e.g., the shield contours; pupils and eyebrows).

Good parallels for this mirror include GERHARD, *ES* I, pl. 45, 5; pl. 46, 3 and 6; BEAZLEY-MAGI, II, pp. 182–183, no. 9; pl. 54; LAMBRECHTS, *Mir. Mus. Royaux*, no. 43 (=Brussels R 1292); DE RIDDER, *Bronzes* II, p. 59 (=Louvre 1798); *AEArq* 33 (1960) fig. 2, 4 (=Madrid 9830); A. EMILIOZZI, *La collezione Rossi Danielli*, Rome 1974, pl. 189; *CSE* Netherlands, nos. 2, 6. Unpublished examples are Florence 609; Karlsruhe F17; F22; F1154.

Compare discussion of date for No. **1**. See also PANDOLFINI in *StEtr* 44 (1976) 247, at no. 56; pl. 51, for a mirror from a tomb at Volsinii, now Vatican 12230, which is identical in subject, similar in style and size, and can be dated by context to *ca.* 300 B.C.

300–250 B.C.

ST. LOUIS, MISSOURI

ST. LOUIS ART MUSEUM

35. Engraved mirror. Figs. 35a–d.

Inv. 155.22. Provenance: unknown. Purchased from Prof. V. G. Simkovitch (New York) in 1922.

C. P. Davis in *Bulletin of the City Art Museum of St. Louis* 9, 1 (1924) 10–11.

Bronze. Intact and in excellent condition except for a few slight cracks at the edge near base of disc. Patina: *Obverse,* good light green patina over a darker blue-green that shows through flaked areas. The handle is well preserved and coated with a fine green patina. *Reverse,* a smooth, light blue area on left is gradually covered by patches of yellow and light green patina. The handle is shinier and more evenly covered.

Measurements: D., 13.1 cm.; Max. H., 27.2 cm.; L. of handle, 11.1 cm.; W. of extension, 3.3 cm.; W. of terminal, 1.2 cm. Weight, 178 gr.

Circular mirror with concave-sided extension and modelled handle cast in one piece. The disc section shows a typical triangular edge profile with a small shelf surrounding the medallion. The edge is undecorated. The central cavity is neatly executed, circular, and 0.12 cm. in diameter. Its use here as part of the design indicating the navel of the seated female is unusual.

Obverse, a deep channel and lightly notched border circle the disc and extension. The area just beneath the extension is decorated with four deep vertical grooves that fan out toward the top. Four short horizontal grooves form a binderlike ornament on the handle. The upper and lower ridges created by the grooves show incised cross-hatching. A single, deep vertical groove runs down the center of the handle toward the animal-head terminal. This is in the form of a ram with modelled horns and features.

Reverse, the handle treatment is virtually identical to the obverse with the exception of the use of small incised arcs to indicate hair on the underside of the animal terminal. The extension is engraved with two stylized acanthus leaves that follow the expanding contours of this area.

Four figures are involved in a dramatic scene, which takes place before an Aeolic/Ionic façade. At the center of the disc is a seated woman, nude except for some drapery wrapped about her right leg. She wears a crown (*cf.* GERHARD, *ES* III, pl. 276, 1–3; pl. 277, 5; KLÜGMANN-KÖRTE, *ES,* pl. 98, 1), a necklace with six round pendants, and high-laced boots. Although she sits with her legs to the left, her arms are extended across the disc. With her left arm she seems to grasp an older male seated at the right; with her right arm she attempts to hold off a younger male who attacks from the left. The young male wears a Phrygian cap, a scabbard strap, a flowing chlamys, and high boots. He grabs the woman by her hair with his left hand and threatens to stab her with the long sword held in his right hand. The older man seated on a decorated stool (perhaps a throne: STEINGRÄBER, type 6) offers an ineffectual gesture of admonition with his extended right hand. He wears a long beard, an unusual hat, and has drapery wrapped about his legs and lower torso. His left hand rests on a knobby staff. Behind the woman we glimpse the head of a third male, who wears a pilos-like hat but with a narrow brim (*cf.* LAMBRECHTS, *Mir. Mus. Royaux,* no. 26 = Brussels R 1276). He appears to restrain the aggressive youth with his extended right arm. A wavy groundline encompasses most of the scene, while a voluminous cable frames the medallion.

The precise mythical episode (if, indeed, this is not a scene from an unrecognized Etruscan legend) is not clear. PRICE, *o.c.,* suggested "Paris, Helen, and Menelaus" or "Hippolytus and Phaedra" but neglected to give his reasons or to cite parallels. "Menelaus threatening Helen" is certainly a possibility. This subject is illustrated on British Museum 627 (=GERHARD, *ES* IV, pl. 398), where the characters are identified by inscription. Menelaus grabs Helen by the hair and threatens her with a drawn sword. She is only partially draped, as on the St. Louis mirror, but clutches the Palladion. The Palladion (or a pillar) appears on several other mirrors where this subject has been recognized (e.g., GERHARD, *ES* IV, pl. 399 = Louvre 1744; pl. 400, 1 = Villa

Giulia 12980), but these could also show "Ajax and Cassandra." In any case, figures similar to the two other males on the St. Louis mirror do not appear on any of these objects.

The old man seated at the right is very similar to one on a mirror (KLÜGMANN-KÖRTE, *ES,* pl. 118) where he is labelled Priumne (Priam), but the type appears elsewhere (e.g., GERHARD, *ES* III, pls. 274, 4; 277, 1) and is probably conventional. For other examples that omit both the seated figure and the Palladion but may still illustrate "Menelaus and Helen," see KLÜGMANN-KÖRTE, *ES,* pl. 116, 1 (=Florence 70533), and *StEtr* 11 (1937) pl. 50, 2 (=Edinburgh 694). Other (less satisfactory) possibilities include "Orestes murdering Clytemnestra" (*cf.* GERHARD, *ES* II, pls. 237–283; KLÜGMANN-KÖRTE, *ES,* pl. 116, 2) or "Odysseus and Circe" (FISCHER-GRAF, V44–46). I know of no Etruscan mirrors that illustrate "Hippolytus and Phaedra."

Stylistically, the engravings may be compared to *CSE* Denmark 1, nos. 1 and 13, but they retain their strong individuality and consistent, confident execution. As a type, the mirror is closely related to *CSE* Netherlands, nos. 7 and 9.

Third century B.C.

36. Engraved mirror. Figs. 36a–d.

Inv. 167.24. Provenance: unknown. Purchased from Kalebdjian Frères (Paris) in 1924. The mirror is almost certainly the one illustrated in GERHARD, *ES* III, pl. 263, 5, and said to have been formerly in the Museo Penacchi at Perugia.

Unpublished.

Bronze. Intact and in good condition. Numerous parallel scratches and deep gouges mar the obverse disc. Patina: *Obverse,* dark brown overall with some patches of dark green patina on the extension and small areas of magenta on the disc. *Reverse,* very similar to the obverse. Some powdery, white incrustations on the handle.

Measurements: D., 10.6 cm.; Max. H., 21.5 cm.; L. of handle, 8.0 cm.; W. of extension, 2.6 cm.; W. of terminal, 1.3 cm. Weight, 239 gr.

Circular mirror with concave-sided extension and massive, modelled handle terminating in a ram's head (*cf.* No. **28**). Disc and handle cast in one piece. The disc section shows that the characteristic medallion shelf has been omitted and the edge profile is not triangular. Deep notches decorate the edge of the disc. The central cavity is 0.1 cm. in diameter.

Obverse, unengraved. Although not as well preserved, the decorative format of the obverse and handle is identical to No. **28**. Minor differences include a smaller, less elaborate execution of the flame motif in the extension and an overall absence of sharp detail in the modelling of the handle.

Reverse, the underside of the ram's-head terminal is decorated with random dots (which continue up the middle of the handle) and a V-shaped double arc. The upper handle, just below the extension, is treated similarly. In many ways this is a simplified version of the format employed on No. **28**. The extension is undecorated.

Four figures appear before a small façade with two Ionic columns. The two central characters are nude. The one on the left stands in three-quarter back view with left arm drawn up and right leg relaxed; the right arm and hand are invisible. This figure, whose sex is impossible to determine, stands on a series of four rounded rocklike forms. The other figure faces forward but turns her head slightly to the right while gesturing with a raised left hand held across her breast. Drapery is tucked between the thighs of this woman. It falls straight to the ground to conceal her right leg. Small clumps of drapery fall from the shoulders of each nude character. Only the second figure has long hair and wears jewelry—bracelets on each wrist and a torque.

The nude figures are flanked by seated males wearing Phrygian caps, laced boots, and some cloth casually draped across their legs. The one on the left rests a lance or staff against his left shoulder; his counterpart on the right holds the hilt of a sword still safely inside its scabbard. This male sits on a small stool (perhaps a diphros but with a leg like that of a kline: STEINGRÄBER, type 3s) with the one visible leg ending in an Ionic capital like those of the background portico. A star, consisting of four petals surrounding a circle, floats beneath the stool. A second star, similar but with four additional circles between the petals, appears in the space between the nude figures' hips (*cf.* the star on No. **8**). A spiky garland with slide binders at top and bottom encloses the scene (*cf.* No. **24**).

The engravings here are very close to those on a mirror reproduced in GERHARD, *ES* III, pl. 263, 5. The minor differences (for example, the omission of the scabbard's lower line) are attributable to the carelessness of the modern artist. GERHARD, p. 295, indicates that the mirror was once in the Museo Penacchi at Perugia. He apparently did not know the mirror's location in 1863. I believe the Perugia mirror eventually found its way to Paris, where it was purchased by the St. Louis Art Museum in 1924.

Five other mirrors are closely related to this example: (1) A mirror from Bolsena (R. BLOCH in *MEFR* 62 [1950]

93, fig. 21) is almost identical in style as well as subject and composition. Small differences include the additional jewelry worn by the nude female and the omission of the star beneath the stool and the staff held by the left male. The right hand and forearm of the left nude are shown. There are also different slide binders for the spiky garland. (2) Villa Giulia 63364 from Vulci (M. T. FALCONI AMORELLI in *ArchCl* 28 [1976] 236; pls. 88, 2; 89) omits both stars and stylistically is close to the Oberlin mirror (our No. **28**). (3) Dresden ZV 30,2 (REBUFFAT, *Miroir,* pl. 87) is very close to the Villa Giulia example. (4) Oberlin 42.122 (No. **28**) is compositionally very close to the St. Louis mirror but substitutes Minerva for the seated male at the right. (5) Paris, Petit Palais DUT 1616 (J. PETIT in *RLouvre* 31, 1 [1982] 27–33, figs. 1–3) omits the stars, has different slide binders, and most significantly, provides a crown for the second figure from the left.

The subject of the St. Louis mirror and examples 1–3 above is presumably the same: two nude males, almost certainly the Dioskouroi, flank two nude females. Only the Oberlin mirror has identifying inscriptions, but here it is clear that the incorporation of Minerva has drastically changed the subject to a Judgment of Paris. BLOCH, *o.c.,* surely is wrong in attempting to interpret the seated male figure on the right of the Bolsena mirror as a hermaphroditic Minerva, thus creating another Judgment of Paris (*cf.* C. PICARD in *RA* 37 [1951] 218).

Moreover, while the sex of the left nudes on mirrors 2–4 cited above is assuredly female (Helen?), it is not easy to be so positive for the St. Louis and Bolsena mirrors. This person could be male, especially on the St. Louis mirror. On still another closely related example where the characters are inscribed (see GERHARD, *ES* IV, pl. 382, 2), this figure, standing in the same effeminate pose, is clearly identified as Ajax (Efas). (Compare similar problems encountered on Copenhagen 2059 = *CSE* Denmark 1, no. 21). But if the figure is male, who is he? He may represent Paris. The nude female on the right would then be Helen; but on the Bolsena mirror she is probably Aphrodite (Turan) because she wears the distinctive kestos often associated with that goddess. See also Brussels R 1288 (= LAMBRECHTS, *Mir. Mus. Royaux,* no. 38) for a related mirror with inscriptions partially preserved. This depicts Minerva and Thalna flanked by two nude youths, perhaps the Dioskouroi.

Only the mirror from Vulci (example 2) has a secure archaeological context; but as Falconi Amorelli has shown, the associated material provides a wide range of possible dates.

Third century B.C.

37. Engraved mirror. Figs. 37a–d.

Inv. 18.26. Provenance: unknown. Purchased from Ercole Canessa (New York) in 1926.

Unpublished.

Bronze. Intact but with several small cracks along the edge and two major cracks at lower disc. Patina: *Obverse,* dark green over lower half of the disc; a shiny light green on the upper half, which is largely covered with encrusted dirt. Good noble light green patina on the extension (where there is some pitting) and upper handle. The middle and lower areas on the handle are a darker green with some dirt and a flaked area. *Reverse,* bright, dark green patina over most of the disc. Some dirt remains around the edge. There are broad areas of pitting on the edge, medallion border, and lower disc.

Measurements: D., 13.6 cm.; Max. H., 27.6 cm.; L. of handle, 10.5 cm.; W. of extension, 3.5 cm.; W. of terminal, 1.2 cm. Weight, 238 gr.

Circular mirror with concave-sided extension and modelled handle cast in one piece. The disc section shows the hooked profile with sharp edge and medallion shelf typical of this type. The central cavity is 0.1 cm. in diameter.

Obverse, the edge is plain. A deep groove surrounds the disc and the unengraved extension. A vertical groove runs down the center of the handle. Near the top, just beneath the extension, are three other grooves that form a floral device. Tiny horizontal incisions decorate the handle's edges. A deer-head terminal forms the standard ornament at the base. Its ears are outlined by punch marks. Long grooves appear on both sides of the handle.

Reverse, the handle decoration is repeated on this side but in simpler form. Fewer grooves ornament the upper portion; the underside of the animal terminal shows a single horizontal groove and is separated from the upper handle by a smaller horizontal groove.

The extension contains three engraved acanthus leaves that unfold into the border and a laurel or olive spray with two berries at the base. The medallion shows a four-figure composition with two women flanked by two men. At the left stands a young man with masses of curly hair. He wears a belted chitoniskos, a chlamys fastened about the neck with a small round button, and high boots. Part of the chlamys is wrapped around his left arm; the rest falls in a series of undulating folds behind his right arm. In his left hand he holds a gnarled club. The second figure, a woman facing left, stands at the center of the disc. Like the man, she places her left hand on her hip. Her right hand is raised to her chin. She wears a belted peplos and perhaps a small diadem; a fibula is visible on her right shoulder. The third figure, also female, stands behind the first woman. Only her head (in left profile) and part of her shoulders are depicted. She wears a hat, perhaps a Phrygian cap, and some drapery. The last character is a nude male, who stands frontally but looks to the left. He wears a chlamys draped over his shoulders, high boots, and a thin fillet about the head. In his left hand he holds a sword in its scabbard. His right hand gently clasps the central woman's left shoulder. Stylized anatomical details on this nude figure are abundant, particularly the *serratus magnus.* Behind the four figures is an architrave decorated with chevrons; above this, a pediment of sorts contains two large leaves and undulating flowers (*cf.* Louvre 1741 = KLÜGMANN-KÖRTE, *ES,* pl. 83, 1, and GERHARD, *ES* III, pl. 272, 1, for similar devices in pediments).

It is impossible to determine the precise identity of the four characters represented on this mirror. The gnarled club, which is the only unconventional attribute shown, is an unlikely indication that the left male is Herakles. There are at least eleven other mirrors that show the same four figures and parallel details of costume, pose, and style: (1) GERHARD, *ES* III, pl. 275, 1 (= Angers, Musée Pincé, 293–13); (2) GERHARD, *ES* III, pl. 275, 2; (3) LAMBRECHTS, *Mir. Mus. Royaux,* no. 26 (= Brussels R 1276); (4) GERHARD, *ES* III, pl. 275A, 1 (= Volterra 914); (5) GERHARD, *ES* III, pl. 276, 5; (6) GERHARD, *ES* IV, pl. 372, 2; (7) D. LEVI in *La Balzana* 1 (1927) 258, fig. 4 (= Grosseto, Museo Civico); (8) REBUFFAT, *Miroir,* pl. 32 (= Biblo. Natl. 1314); (9) GERHARD, *ES* I, pl. 59, 4; (10) M. T. FALCONI AMORELLI in *ArchCl* 27 (1975) 56, no. 2 (= Tolentino, Museo Civico); (11) G. LLOYD-MORGAN in *PBSR* 43 (1975) pl. II (= Birmingham 153'48). None of the figures on these mirrors carries a gnarled club. However, a related mirror in the De Menil Collection (Houston, no. 74.14DJ = DE GRUMMOND, *Guide,* p. 160, fig. 6) shows the left male carrying a club. In this case, the subject is the Judgment of Paris and there are three, not two, females. Another mirror of related type and style may also show a Judgment of Paris with the sole male figure carrying a club (see GERHARD, *ES* II, pl. 187).

The St. Louis mirror belongs to a large group characterized by the distinctive handle ornament, extension design, and four-figure composition enclosed by a leafy border. In addition to the examples listed above, the following stylistic parallels should be cited: (1–2) LAMBRECHTS, *Mir. Mus. Royaux,* nos. 3 and 39 (= Brussels R 1253 and R 1289); (3) *CSE* Netherlands, no. 4; (4) *CSE* Bologna I, no. 17; (5–7) GERHARD, *ES* II, pl. 186; III, pl. 272, 1; IV, pl. 369, 2.

Third Century B.C.

TOLEDO, OHIO

TOLEDO MUSEUM OF ART

38. Unengraved mirror. Figs. 38a–b.

Inv. 11.46. Provenance: unknown. Given by Arthur F. Bissel, New York, in 1911.

Unpublished.

Bronze. Intact and in excellent condition. Patina: *Obverse,* the disc is covered evenly with cuprite and some traces of azurite. There are a few areas of heavy corrosion at the top of the disc. The upper handle and lower part of the extension reveal smooth, shiny bronze. *Reverse,* similar to the obverse but with heavier corrosion at top of disc and a less uniform green overall. There are a few patches of shiny bronze on the extension and upper handle.

Measurements: Horizontal D., 13.6 cm.; Vertical D., 15.2 cm.; Max. H., 26.5 cm.; H. of handle, 10.5 cm.; W. of extension, 3.2 cm.; W. top of handle, 2.0 cm.; W. of animal terminal, 0.5 cm. Weight, 230 gr.

Piriform mirror having concave-sided extension with sharp points and a handle terminating in a very stylized animal head. The disc and handle are cast in one piece. The edge is undecorated. The section is slightly convex, and there is a small hook in profile on the obverse.

Obverse, a shallow groove surrounds the disc and extension. There is a typical beaded border which parallels the outer edge of this groove. The extension and handle are smooth and undecorated except for two deep lines forming an engraved "V" just above the animal terminal. The terminal itself is very small and abstract. It probably represents a deer and perhaps the engraved V marks the extended, long ears of this creature.

Reverse, completely unornamented. There is no central cavity.

The characteristic piriform shape and section of this mirror associate it with Praenestine workshops. A fair number of mirrors excavated at (or connected by style with) Praeneste are undecorated (see comments for No. **23**). The unusually diminished terminal as well as the engraved "ears"

on the obverse are paralleled by Brussels R 1295 (=LAMBRECHTS, *Mir. Mus. Royaux,* no. 46).

Probably *ca.* 300–275 B.C.

39. Engraved mirror. Figs. 39a–d.

Inv. 80.1340. Provenance: Praeneste, discovered in 1868. Formerly in the collections of Count Michal Tyszkiewicz, Antonio Sambon, Benjamin Fillon, and S. Schweizer. Given to the museum by Edward Drummond Libbey in 1980.

W. Helbig, *BullInst* (1869) 14; *MonIst* 9 (1869) pl. 7, 3; H. HEYDEMANN, *AnnInst* (1869) 198; *Ephemeris Epigraphica* 1 (1872) p. 12, no. 18; R. GARRUCI, *Sylloge inscriptionum Latinarum* . . . (1875–77) no. 530; O. RAYET, *GazBA* 18, (1878) pp. 367, 370; *CII, App.,* no. 475; *Collection B. Fillon, Catalogue de vente* (Paris 1882) p. 26, no. 11; ill. on p. 27; *CIL* 14 (1887) p. 473, no. 4094; E. LATTES, *Le iscrizioni paleolatine* . . . (Milan 1892) no. 113; KLÜGMANN-KÖRTE, *ES,* pp. 113–114; pl. 90; O. ROSSBACH in *Festschrift für Otto Benndorf* (Vienna 1898), p. 150; F. BEHN, *Die Ficoronische Cista* (Rostock 1907), pp. 63–64; MATTHIES, *PS,* p. 73, fig. 12; *CIL* I, pt. 2, fasc. 1 (1918), p. 428, no. 548; GIGLIOLI, *AE,* p. 57; pl. 304, 3; L. MARCHESE, *StEtr* 18 (1944) p. 57, fig. 2; BEAZLEY, *EVP,* p. 58; T. P. HOWE, *AJA* 61(1957) 344, n. 20, pl. 102, fig. 3; G. MANSUELLI, *EAA* 1 (1958) p. 334, fig. 477; M. SAPELLI, *Acme* 28 (1975) pp. 243–244, fig. 12; C. MACCABRUNI, *NumAntCl* 6 (1977) pp. 53–71; pls. 1–3; *Sotheby Auction Catalogue* (London, 15 July 1980), pp. 54–55, no. 99; Toledo Museum of Art, *The Museum Collects: Treasures by Sculptors and Craftsmen* (7 December 1980–25 January 1981), pp. 12–13; H. WEIS, *AJA* 86 (1982) pp. 33–34, no. 6; G. BECKEL, *LIMC* I (1982), p. 740, no. 13; E. RICHARDSON, *ArchN* 13, 3/4 (1984) 57–67, figs. 1–4.

Bronze. Intact and in excellent condition. Patina: *Obverse,* a very fine, smooth, light green patina covers the disc. There are some minor scratches and areas of pitting. The handle, which has a dark green patina, shows only small areas of uneven corrosion. The extension ornament has recently been infilled with white paint. *Reverse,* the smooth surface shows evidence of an earlier mechanical cleaning of the disc. There are areas of azurite, some malachite, but mostly cuprite deposits. Large patches on the left side of disc are shiny bronze. Corrosion products around the edge are higher and less smooth than those of the disc. An earlier wax coating has been removed; the mirror was recently lacquered with Acryloix B–72 and the engravings (which showed smooth corrosion products) have been infilled with white paint.

Measurements: Horizontal D., 16.9 cm.; Vertical D., 18.3 cm.; Max. H., 31.1 cm.; H. of handle, 12.0 cm.; W. of extension, 4.4 cm.; W. top of handle, 2.7 cm.; W. of animal terminal, 1.2 cm. Weight, 655 gr.

Piriform mirror having an extension with concave sides, pronounced extension points, and a handle terminating is a deer's head. Disc and handle cast in one piece. The slightly convex edge is decorated with an ovolo and bead design in relief. These two elements are separated by a tiny torus moulding; the whole is about 0.4 cm. high. Compare No. **20** and LAMBRECHTS, *Mir. Mus. Royaux,* no. 36, p. 226. The section is typical of Praenestine mirrors (*cf.* Nos. **13, 14, 20, 21, 23, 38**). The central cavity is 0.3 cm. in diameter. There is also a smaller, uneven cavity 0.2 cm. in diameter just below it. A similar situation exists on another Praenestine mirror, Brussels R 1261 = LAMBRECHTS, *Mir. Mus. Royaux,* no. 11; see also p. 75.

Obverse, a delicate beaded border, part of the edge decoration, ornaments the unengraved disc and continues down the sides of the extension and handle to the base of the terminal. Each of the handle's four sides is a long, concave panel edged with a deep groove. The terminal, the best-preserved and best-executed example of the mirrors treated in this fascicle, shows an intricately engraved and modelled deer's head. Details such as the bulging eyes, long ears, and round muzzle are enhanced by delicate engraved lines. A series of uniformly drawn arcs covers the head and neck to indicate the animal's mottled skin. Two small engraved circles in front of the ears represent the deer's incipient horns. For this unusual detail, see LAMBRECHTS, *Mir. Mus. Royaux,* nos. 9, 11, and 34.

Major decoration on the obverse is concentrated in the elaborate engravings of the extension and lower disc. Here we see an elegant palmette with six curved leaves and a central stem, which appears to be a floral bud. Two small circular buds or blossoms flank this central stem. All of these elements rise from a pistil flanked by small, horizontally disposed volutes. A pair of large serrated leaves enclose the palmette; smaller leaflike elements frame the bottom volutes. A Praenestine mirror in the Birmingham City Museum (no. 447′61) shows a virtually identical motif: see G. LLOYD-MORGAN in *PBSR* 43 (1975) 78–79; pl. 1. The "background" of this design is picked out by numerous round punch marks. Compare the similar treatment on Brussels R 1283 (= LAMBRECHTS, *Mir. Mus. Royaux,* no. 33, p. 206).

Reverse, the border consists of an undulating ivy vine with trilobed leaves (all of which point down) and round berries. The vines spring from the points of the extension and partially enclose two swimming dolphins (*cf.* GERHARD, *ES* II, pl. 139). The vines reach to the top of the disc, where they frame a small female head shown frontally. An exergue is created by a wide egg-and-dart frieze (*cf.* GERHARD, *ES* II, pl. 163; III, pl. 251; IV, pls. 337, 1 [= Villa Giulia 12978] and 377). At its base, between the leaping dolphins, is a large palmette with flanking volutes; this is essentially an inverted version of the device seen on the obverse.

Three male figures appear in the medallion. On the left a nude youth stands with his back toward us. (For the pose, *cf.* KLÜGMANN-KÖRTE, *ES,* pl. 91, 1.) He holds a spear on his left shoulder and carries a draped chlamys over his left arm; he reaches for (or holds?) a pilos in his right hand. Beside the right shoulder and running vertically from top to bottom is the following inscription:

$$CΛST o R$$

c a s t o r

A large bearded man is bound to a tall tree trunk at the medallion's center. He faces right, is bent at the waist, and appears in three-quarter view. His hair and beard are short; the eyebrows are abundant. Numerous small parallel lines model the musculature of his powerful body; these also appear on the other figures but to a lesser degree. The tree's bark is indicated with wavy vertical lines. The second identifying inscription runs from left to right in the space to the right of the central figure's hips:

$$AMV(o S$$

a m u c o s

The third figure stands in profile at the right. He faces the bound Amykos and holds his right hand near the king's shoulder. The young god, who wears a laurel crown in his long hair, holds a spear or long staff in his left hand. He wears boots and a himation draped over his left shoulder. Above his head, running left to right, is the third identifying inscription:

$$ΓO LoV(ξς$$

p o l o u c e s

Several irregular shapes indicate rocks on or before which the figures stand. At the extreme right of the medallion is a lion-head spout from which issues the waters of a natural spring.

The mirror illustrates the Dioskouroi (Castor and Pollux-Polydeukes) with King Amykos. This story of the Argonauts' encounter with Amykos, King of the Bebrykes, is frequently presented on engraved mirrors and cistae. The relationships are discussed by many of the authors cited above, especially Matthies, Marchese, Beazley, Maccabruni, and Beckel. In addition, see T. DOHRN, *Die Ficoronische Ciste* (Berlin 1972), and FOERST, *GPC,* pp. 46–50.

Despite the proliferation of sensuous ornament, the composition of this mirror's medallion is relatively simple. A central figure, vertically disposed, is flanked by two other vertical figures. One nicety of design is the introduction of a back view (Castor) juxtaposed with the much more common three-quarter view (Polouces). The engraving is very fine, especially for the ornaments on each side. There is some hesitancy in the execution of portions of the figures and their drapery.

About 300 B.C.

ADDENDA

The following mirrors were only recently acquired by midwestern museums or brought to my attention. Some had been lost, while others were mistakenly classified as Greek or Egyptian. In an attempt to make this fascicle as complete as possible, I have decided to include them, although several will be published elsewhere in more extended form. Information for some of these, especially Nos. **42–45**, is incomplete; chemical analyses are available for only two, Nos. **40** and **41**. Too late for inclusion here is an important mirror recently acquired by the University of Wisconsin, Madison (Inv. No. 1986.24). It will appear in my article for the *Bulletin of the Elvehjem Museum of Art* (1987).

BLOOMINGTON, INDIANA

INDIANA UNIVERSITY ART MUSEUM

40. Unengraved mirror. Figs. 40a–b.

Inv. 62.117.110. Provenance: unknown. Gift of Burton Y. Berry.

Unpublished.

Bronze. Intact and in good condition. A few recent scratches mar both sides; several large round pits on the reverse. Patina: both sides have an overall brown-green or dark green patina with a few patches of shiny bronze showing through it. The obverse, which is relatively free of large pits, shows striated bands of small eruptions.

Measurements: D., 14.6 cm.; Max. H., 19.9 cm.; L. of tang, 5.4 cm.; W. of extension, 2 cm. Weight, 714.3 gr.

Mirror with elliptical disc and tapering tang cast in one piece. The disc shows a perfectly flat profile with slightly rounded edges. The disc is thicker than most mirrors (0.5 cm.), which accounts for its heaviness. However, *CSE* Bologna II, no. 3, has a similar section and is almost as thick (0.4 cm.). The extension is small with convex sides; the tang tapers to a rounded point. There is neither a central cavity nor engraved or modelled decoration on this mirror.

A close parallel for shape and size is BEAZLEY-MAGI, pl. 53, no. 15, with two related examples (also in the Vatican) mentioned on p. 186.

Probably early fifth century B.C.

CHICAGO, ILLINOIS

ART INSTITUTE OF CHICAGO

41. Engraved mirror. Figs. 41a–e.

Inv. 1984.1341. Provenance: unknown. Formerly in the R. Zietz collection, London. Purchased through the Katherine Adler Fund from Michael Ward, Inc. in 1984.

Unpublished. Michael Ward, Inc., *First Exhibition 1983,* no. 1 (color photo of reverse); R. DE PUMA, *Art Institute of Chicago Museum Studies* 14 (1987), forthcoming.

Bronze. Intact except for broken tang and in fair condition. A deep crack on the upper right of obverse disc; a smaller crack appears to the left of extension (reverse). Portions of the lower left edge are heavily corroded and separating. Patina: *Obverse,* a hard, smooth, light green or blue-green surface is spotted by several patches of heavy corrosion, especially around the edge of the disc. In some areas (bottom and left side) this is combined with encrusted dirt. Pitted areas are prominent near the center. *Reverse,* very fine, smooth, and hard blue-green patina over entire surface. There are small patches of minor eruptions on the engraved figures, but only one area, the lower right edge, is severely obscured by corrosion. The detail (Fig. 41e) illustrates excellently the so-called dendritic formations characteristic of bronzes that have not been reheated after casting. For other examples, see F. C. THOMPSON, *Numismatic Chronicle* 6th ser., 16 (1956) 332–336, ills. 7–9, and B. VON FREYTAG GEN. LÖRINGHOFF in U. HAUSMANN, *Der Tübinger Waffenläufer = Tübinger Studien zur Archäologie und Kunstgeschichte* 4 (1977) 45–48, pl. 10, 3–4.

Measurements: D., 15.1 cm.; Max. H., 16.6 cm.; Pres. L. of tang, 0.9 cm.; W. of extension, 1.9 cm.; W. of tang, 0.7 cm. Weight, 353 gr.

Circular mirror with small, convex-sided extension and a tapering tang. The disc section is very slightly convex on the reflecting side. The rim (0.45 cm. thick) is elegantly modelled with an ovolo border, a simple horizontal line, and a beaded border. No. **15** has the same design and section; *cf. CSE* Denmark 1, no. 26, for a similar mirror. There is no central cavity.

Obverse, the extension ornament consists of an elaborately engraved series of spirals symmetrically arranged on either side of a triangle. A somewhat similar motif appears on *CSE* Bologna I, no. 10. The fine beaded border surrounds the disc and extension.

Reverse, the medallion is filled with a representation of Eos holding the body of Memnon (see No. **15**). The goddess stands on a short groundline decorated with an ovolo frieze. Her right foot is shown in profile, while her left foot is slightly raised and seen from above. She wears a chiton and voluminous mantle, the hems of which are ornamented carefully with rows of tiny, square punch marks (*cf.* Nos. **15, 34**). The drapery folds are indicated by cursory arcs. Her head appears in right profile with the hair indicated by a series of nearly parallel, wavy verticals. She wears a fillet and necklace or collar, also decorated with square punch marks. Her hands and feet are crudely rendered and contrast sharply with the delicate and complicated treatment of her wings where numerous fine strokes enliven each feather.

The goddess holds the naked body of her dead or dying son. There is little anatomical rendering—the abdominal muscles, the shins, and the awkwardly placed genitals. His profile and hair are very similar to those of his mother. Perhaps he is still holding or has just dropped his sword. His crested helmet, elaborated with punch marks, falls dramatically from his head.

The disc is surrounded by an ivy leaf border which sprouts from the extension area. This is decorated with an engraved volute cluster tucked below the groundline. Engravings are generally firm and confident. There are a few omissions: the lower left feather of Eos' left wing does not continue behind Memnon's helmet nor do the lines of her drapery; some lines indicating the garment hems are not consistent.

The general quality of the engravings may be compared to Brussels R 1270 from Viterbo (see LAMBRECHTS, *Mir. Mus. Royaux,* no. 20) and, perhaps, to a mirror formerly on the Swiss market, *Münzen und Medaillen, Sonderliste J* (1968) no. 31.

About 470–450 B.C.

CINCINNATI, OHIO

CINCINNATI ART MUSEUM

42. Engraved mirror. Figs. 42a–c.

Inv. 1884.194. Provenance: "Found in a tomb near Pales-trina." Acquired from Augusto Castellani in 1884 and given to the Museum by the Women's Art Museum Association.

Unpublished.

Bronze. Intact except for broken tang. Patina: very heavily cor-roded with dense incrustations on all surfaces.

Measurements: D., 16.5 cm.; Max. H., 18.8 cm.; L. of tang, 2.2 cm. Weight, 474.45 gr.

Circular mirror with tapering tang but no extension. The section is typical of early tang mirrors and shows a slight concavity on the reverse with a round thickening of the rim. There is no central cavity visible.

There are no signs of any decoration on the obverse, but traces of engraved designs are barely discernible on the reverse. These are presented, tentatively, in the accompany-ing sketch (Fig. 42a) and seem to indicate that the reverse is decorated with a Siren. This subject makes the mirror very interesting because only one other mirror is known with the same subject: GERHARD, *ES* IV, pl. 429, 2, formerly in Berlin but now lost. According to Gerhard's drawing, that mirror had lost its extension and tang and the design is somewhat different.

MAYER-PROKOP, *Griffspiegel* S17, p. 21, also discusses the Berlin mirror and offers comments on a number of other Sirens in Etruscan art on pp. 72–75. One may also note the exergue Siren on Bologna 1070: *CSE* Bologna I, no. 40 and p. 56.

Probably *ca.* 500–460 B.C.

43. Unengraved mirror. Figs. 43a–b.

Inv. 1884.195. Provenance: Palestrina. Acquired from Augusto Castellani in 1884 and given to the Museum by the Women's Art Museum Association.

Unpublished.

Bronze. Intact except for a fragment missing from the upper edge of the disc and some flakes missing from the rim. The number 4 written in blue on the obverse follows Castellani's ordering of the objects in this group. Patina: uniformly dark green and powdery. The handle is in better condition generally than the disc.

Measurements: Horizontal D., 13.1 cm.; Vertical D., 14.1 cm.; Max. H., 21.3 cm.; H. of handle, 6.4 cm.; W. of extension, 2.8 cm.; W. top of handle, 1.6 cm.; W. of terminal, 1.1 cm. Weight, 78.4 gr.

Piriform mirror with concave-sided extension and short handle terminating in a very abstracted animal head. The section is very thin, with a slight concavity but no thick-ening of the rim. There is no central cavity.

The only decoration on this mirror is found on the handle. Just above the stylized animal-head terminal are four parallel, horizontal lines on the obverse and two on the reverse. These seem to act as a collar for the head, which is enlivened simply by two deep grooves (hinting at ears) and a horizontal line across its middle.

Third century B.C.

44. Unengraved mirror. Figs. 44a–b.

Inv. 1884.196. Provenance: Palestrina. Acquired from Augusto Castellani in 1884 and given to the Museum by the Women's Art Museum Association.

Unpublished.

Bronze. Intact except for the right extension point on the obverse. A large crack at the top of the disc has caused the rim to separate from the disc. Patina: light green on both sides but largely obscured by heavy incrustations of corrosion and dirt.

Measurements: Horizontal D., 13.4 cm.; Vertical D., 15.2 cm.; Max. H., 24.8 cm.; H. of handle, 9.3 cm.; W. of extension, 5 cm.; W. top of handle, 3.2 cm.; W. of animal terminal, 1.1 cm. Weight, 242.7 gr.

Piriform mirror with wide, concave-sided extension and handle terminating in a deer's head. The section is thin and slightly curved, with a high rim set at a sharp angle to the disc. A central cavity is not visible now.

There are two areas of decoration. The exterior rim is given an incised ovolo border which surrounds the disc but ends at the points of the extension. The handle terminal is a modelled deer's head with eyes and ears indicated on the obverse; the reverse side is flat and unmodelled.

In size and shape the mirror is roughly similar to No. **38** but not as refined. Parallels for this Praenestine type include examples published in *MonAL* 20 (1910) col. 108, fig. 78, and by A. EMILIOZZI, *Coll. Rossi Danielli,* nos. 587–588.

Probably 300–250 B.C.

45. Fragmentary engraved(?) mirror. Figs. 45a–b.

Inv. 1947.271. Provenance: unknown. Given by Millard F. and Edna F. Shelt in 1947.

Unpublished.

Bronze. Fragmentary handle mirror with handle, extension, and portions of the disc missing. Patina: all surfaces are heavily corroded.

Measurements: D., 13.3 cm. Pres. weight, 237.4 gr.

Fragmentary handle mirror. The section appears typical, with a slight concavity and a thickened triangular hook at the rim. A central cavity is not visible now.

It is likely that this mirror was originally engraved, but until it is cleaned, we can only speculate on the possible subject. One statistically promising subject is the Dioskouroi (*cf.* Nos. **9** and **22**, which are close in size and shape).

Third century B.C.?

FIGURES

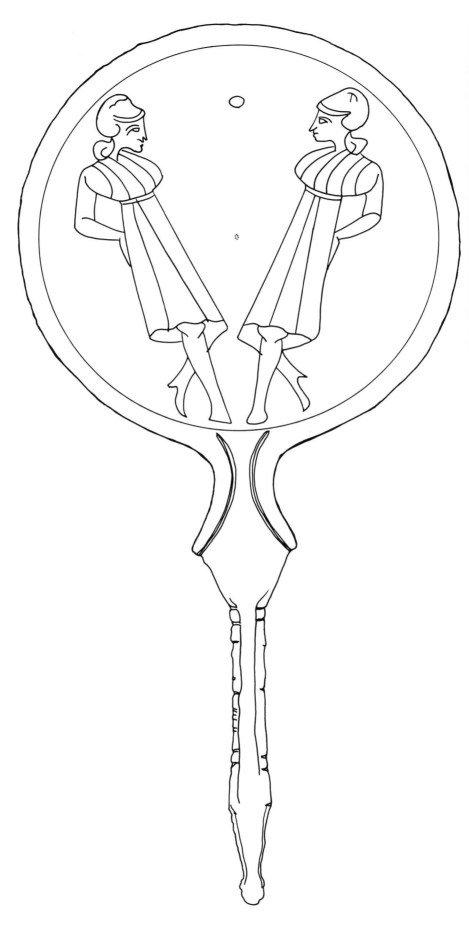

1a

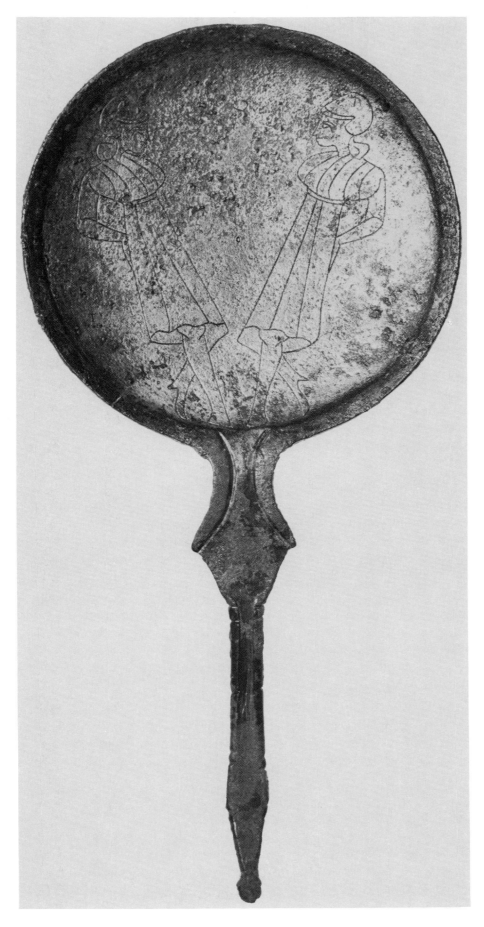

1b

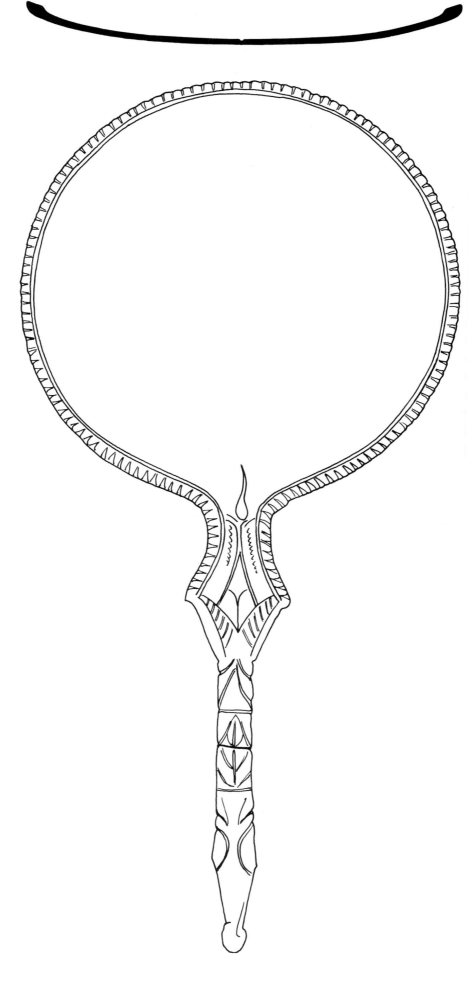

1c

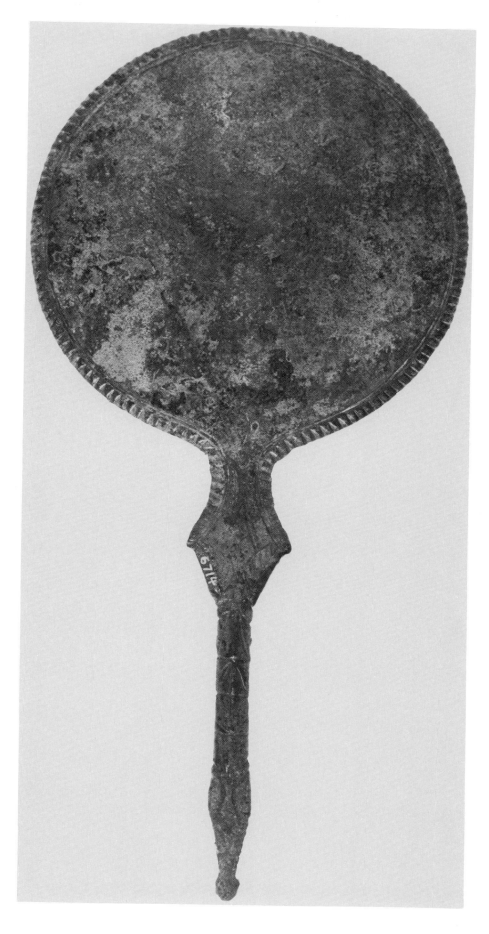

1d

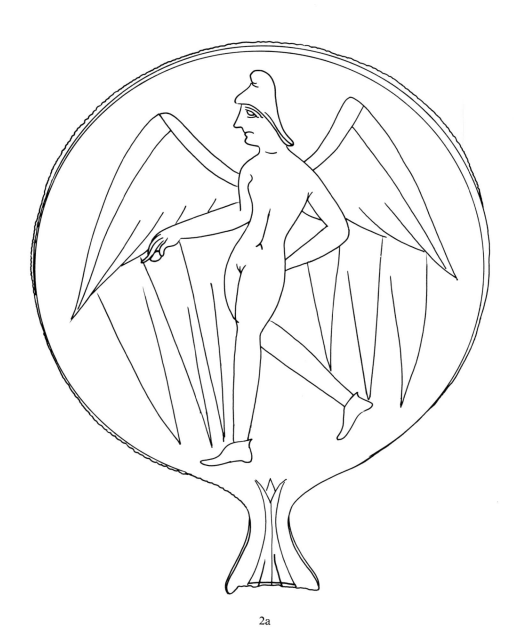

2a

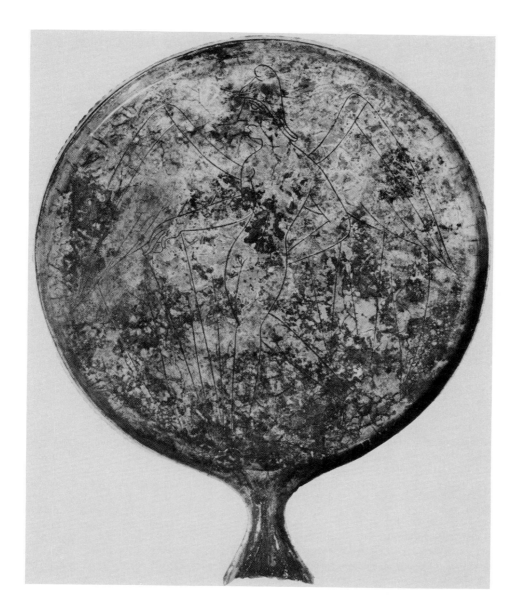

2b

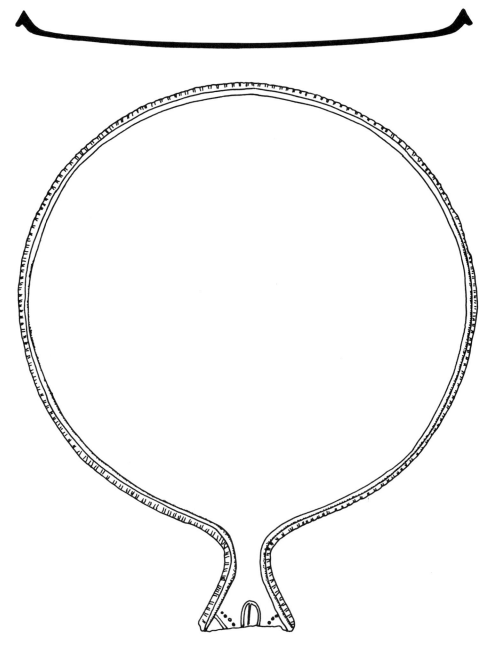

2c

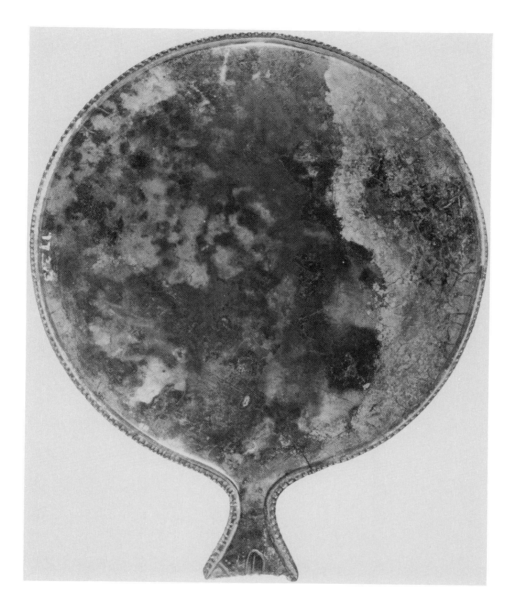

2d

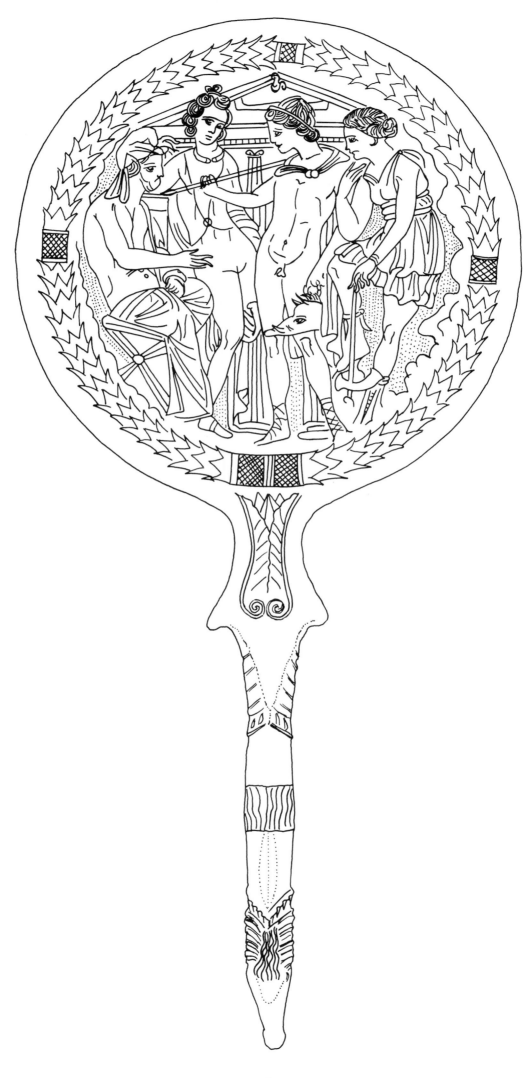

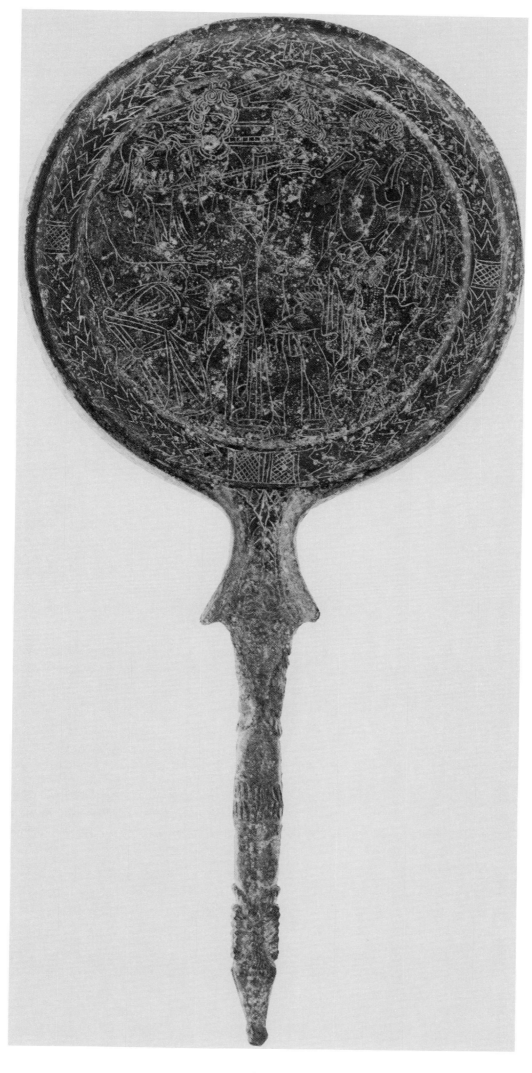

74

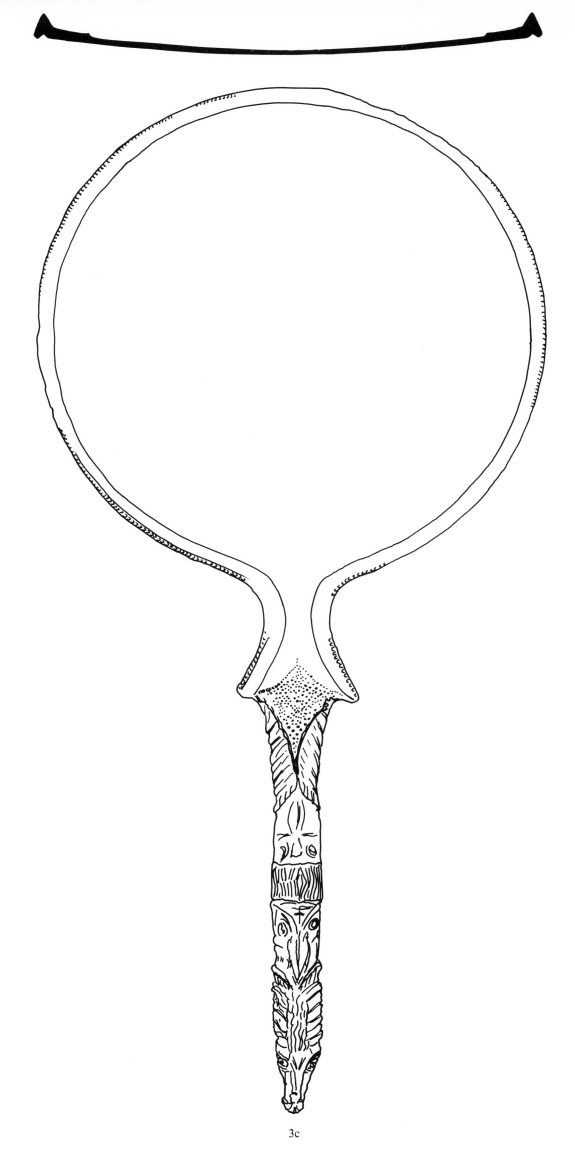

3c

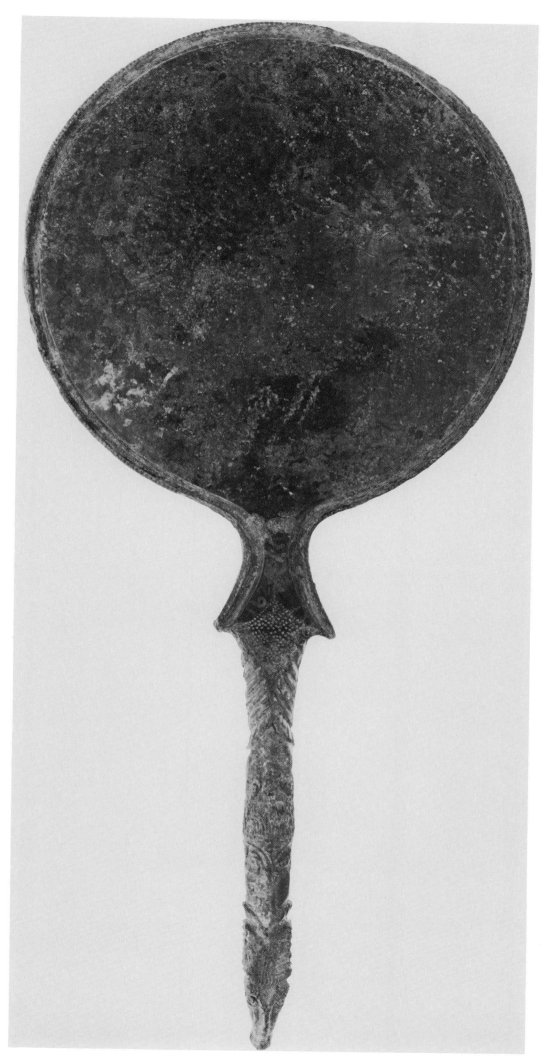

3d

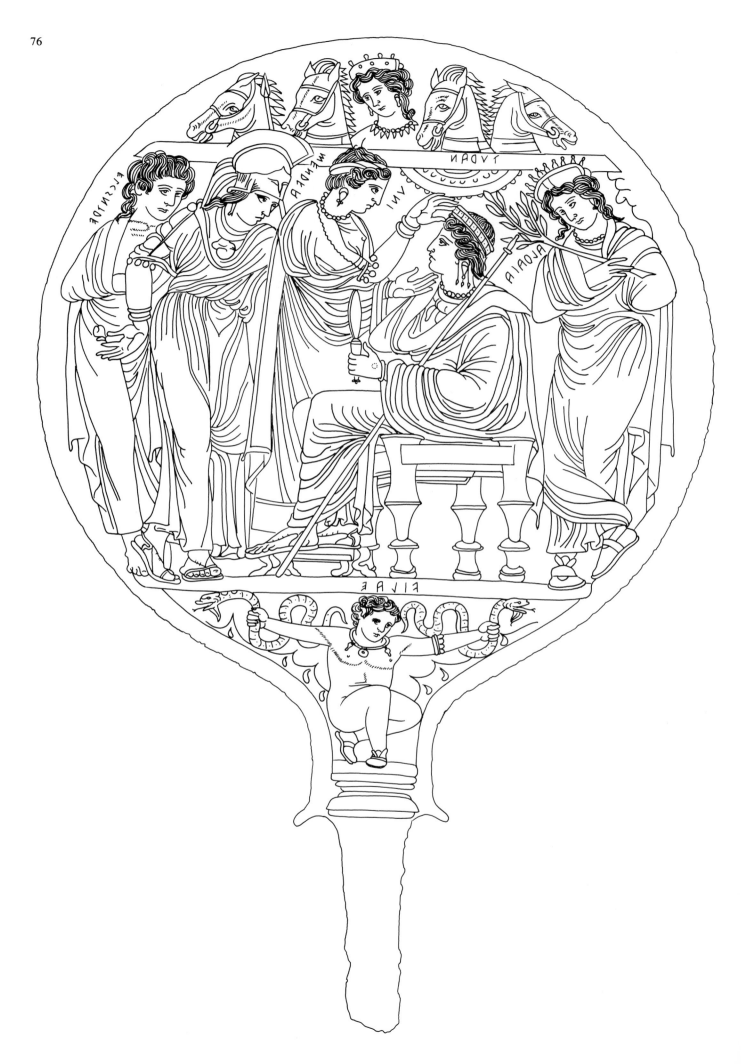

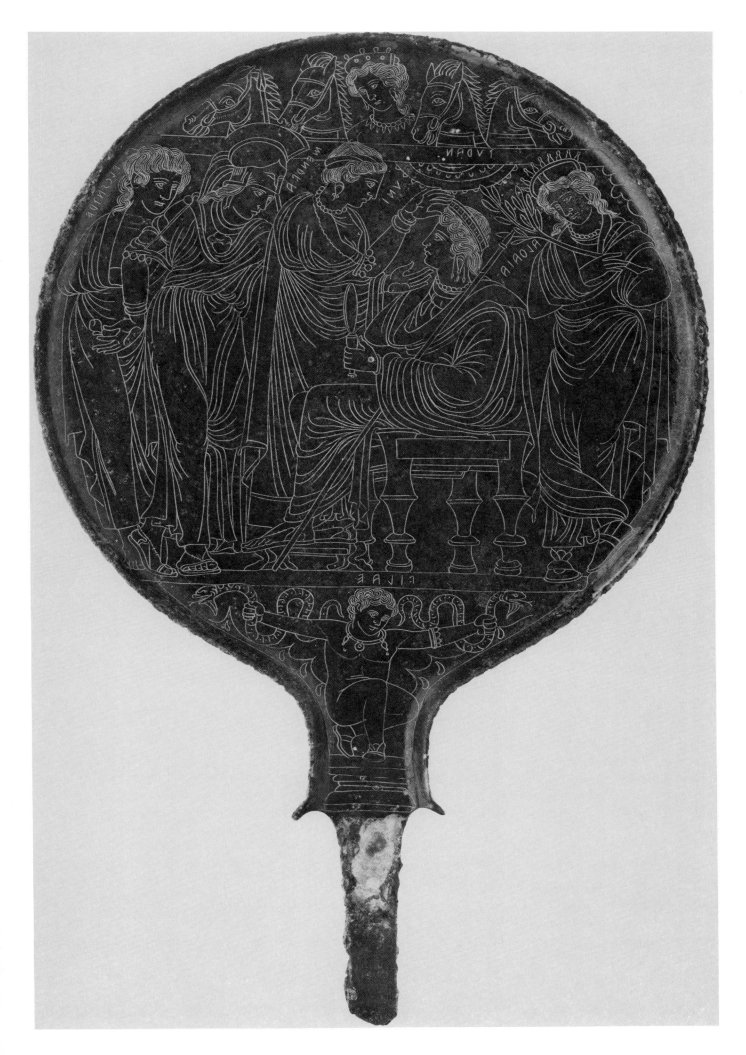

4b

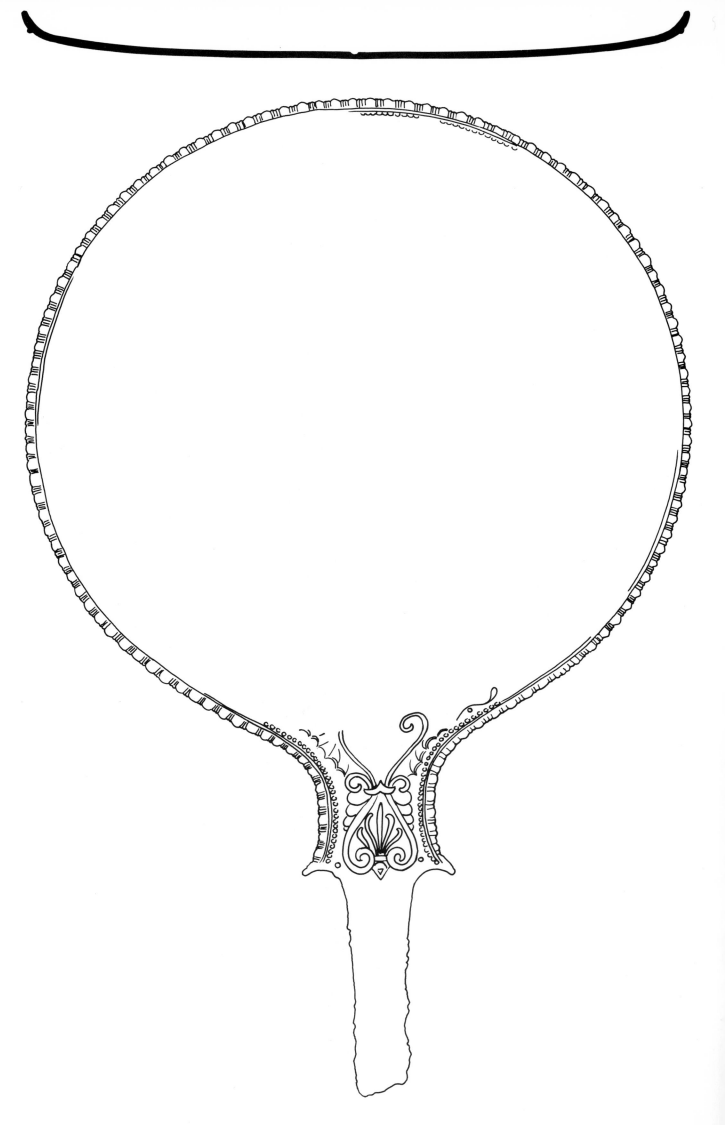

4c

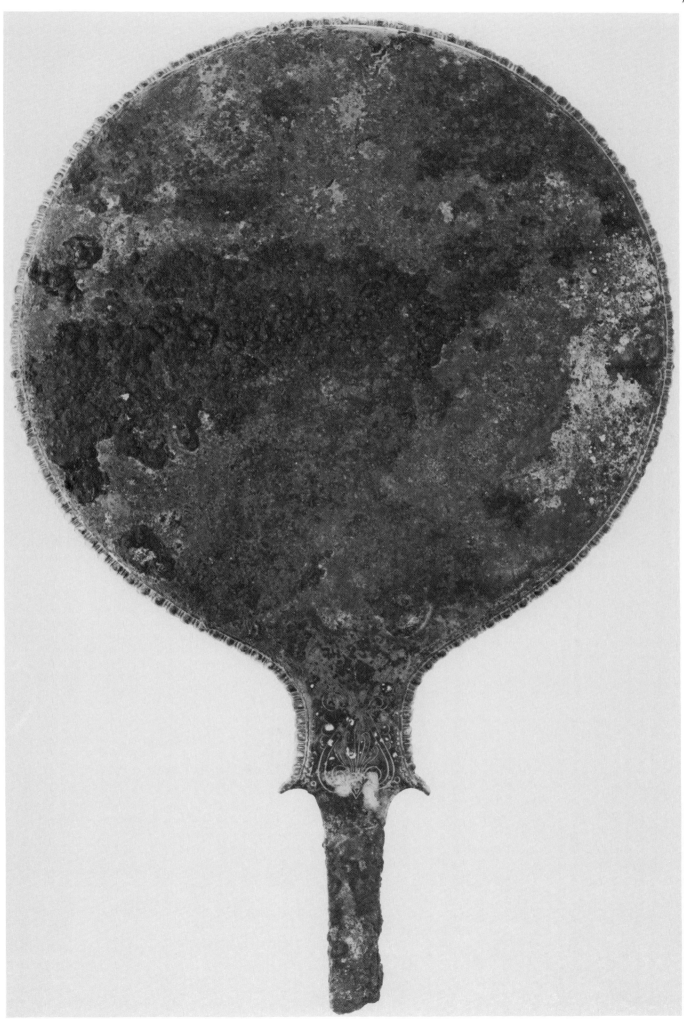

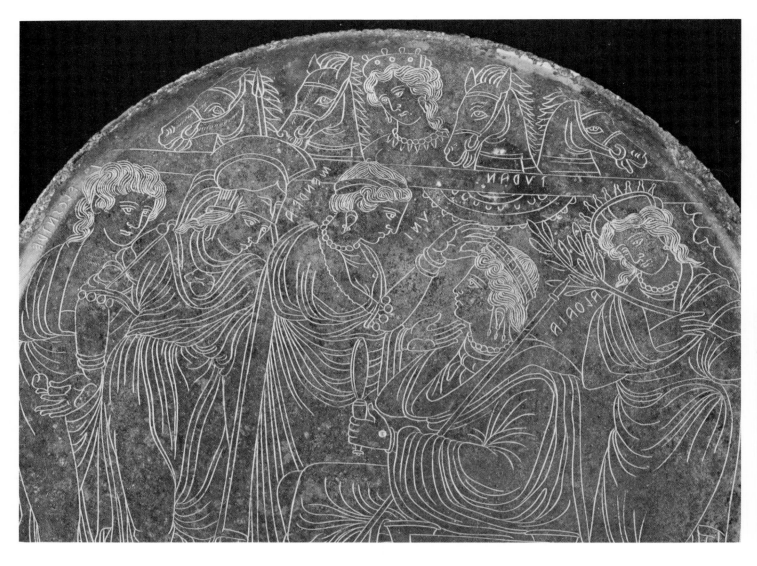

4e

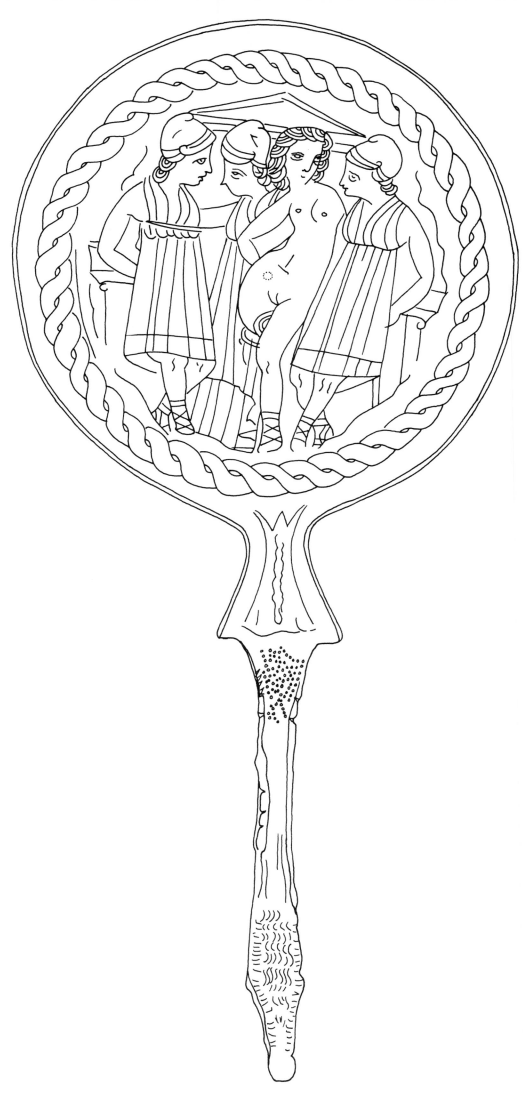

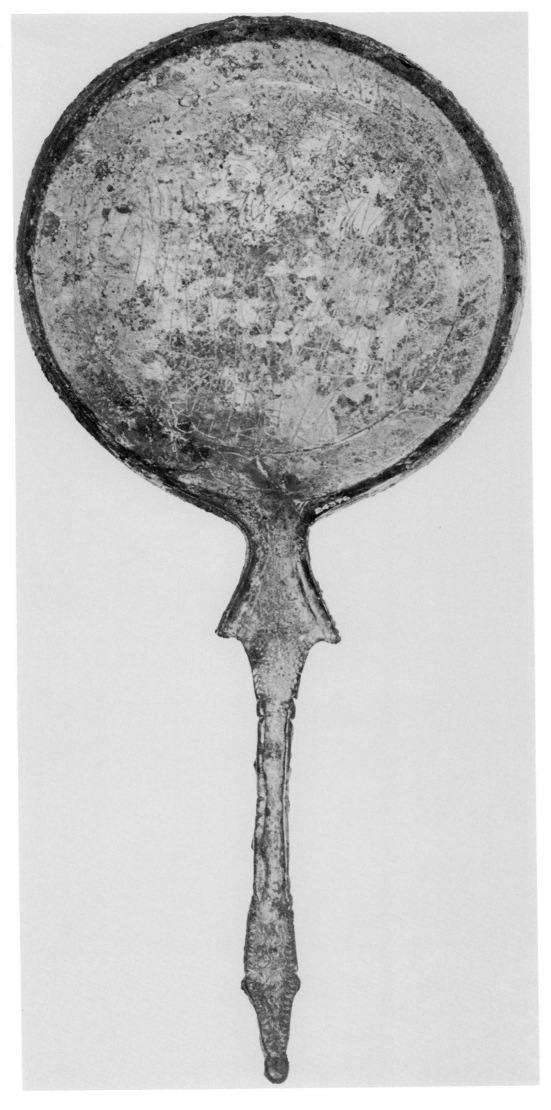

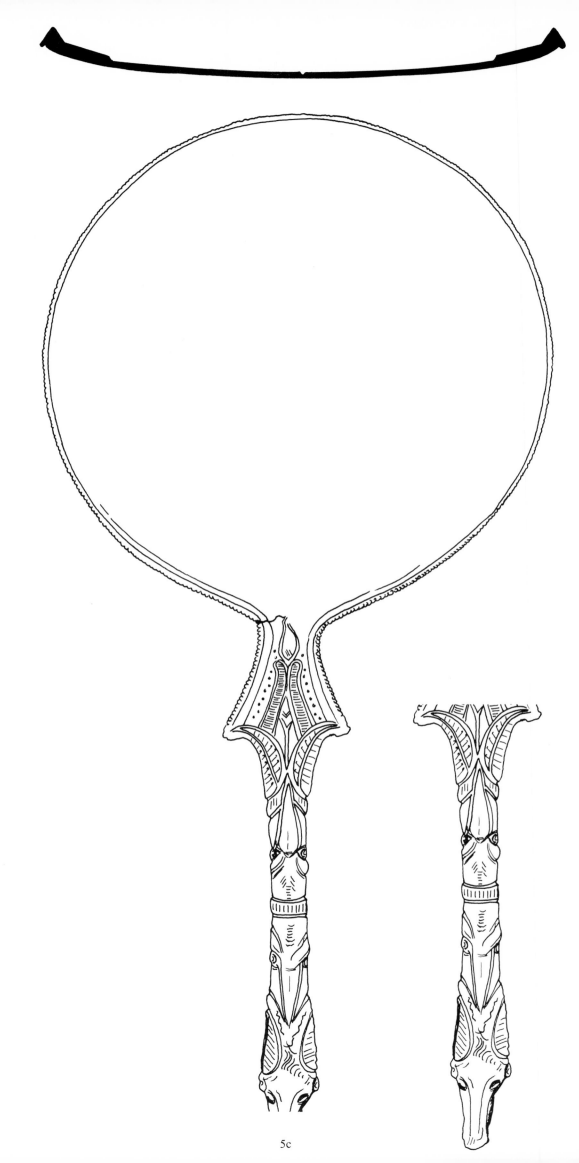

5c

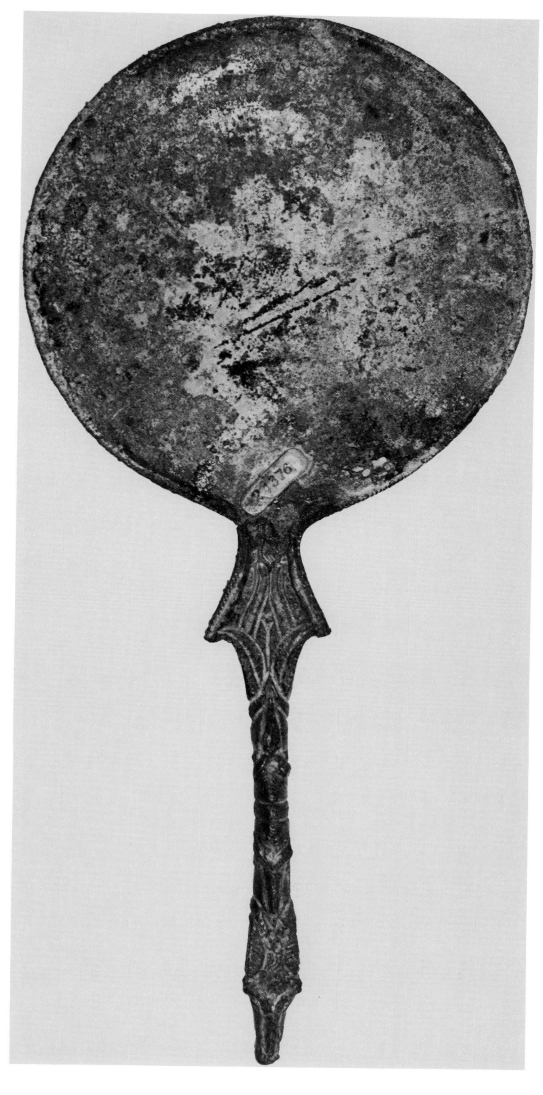

5d

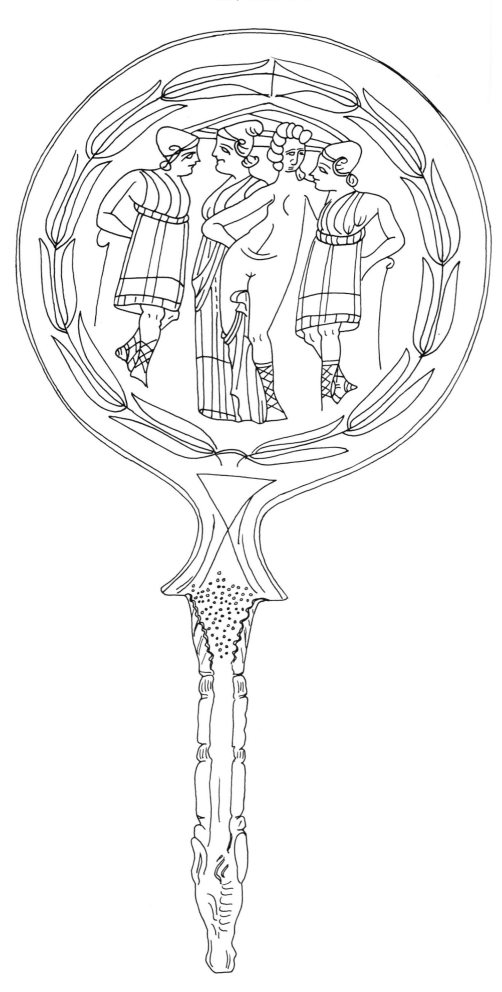

6a

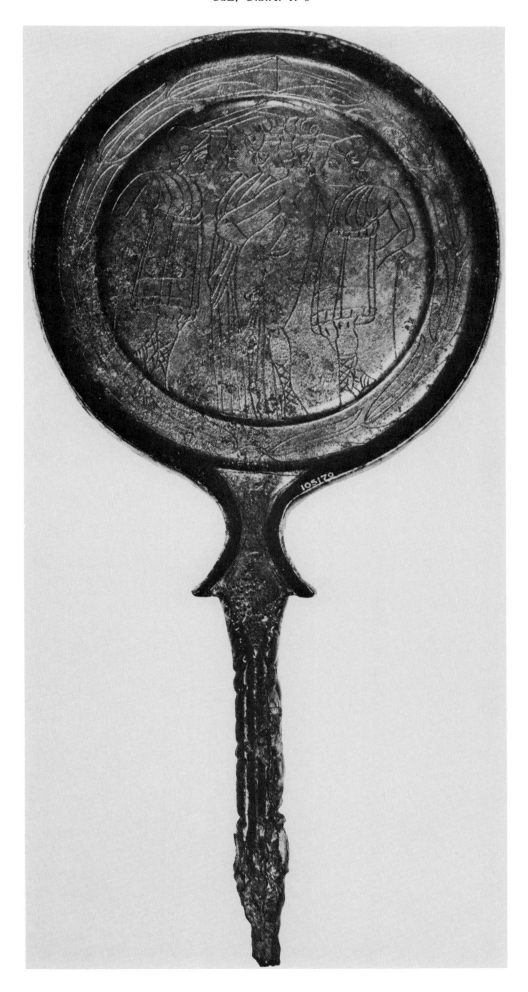

6b

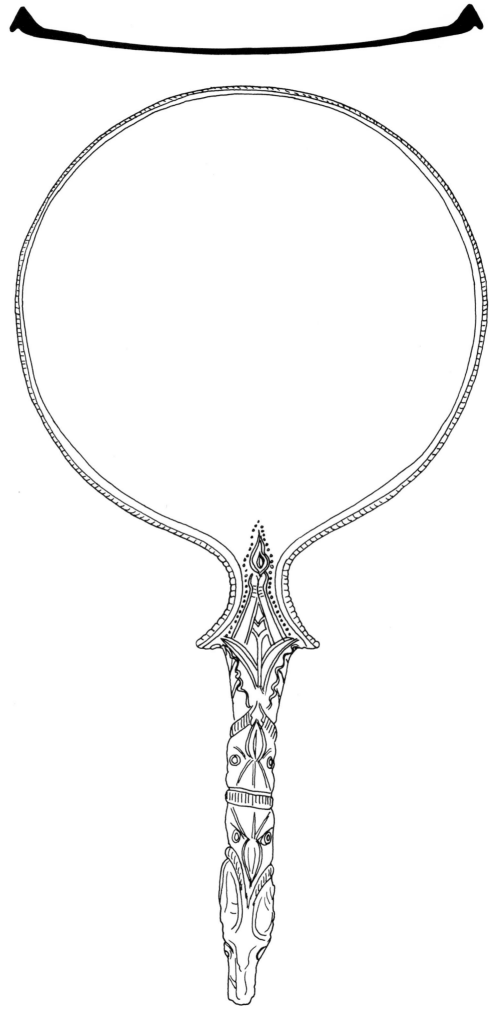

6c

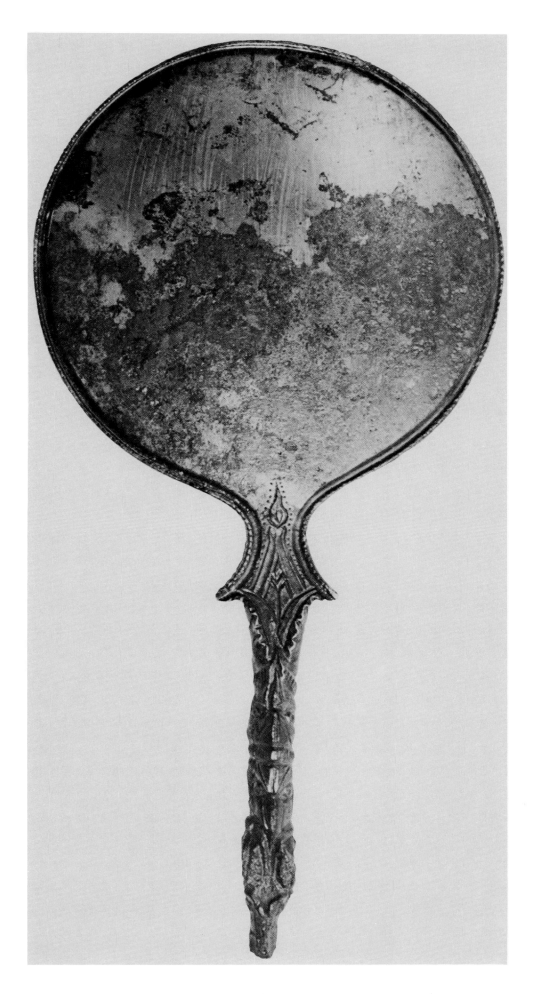

6d

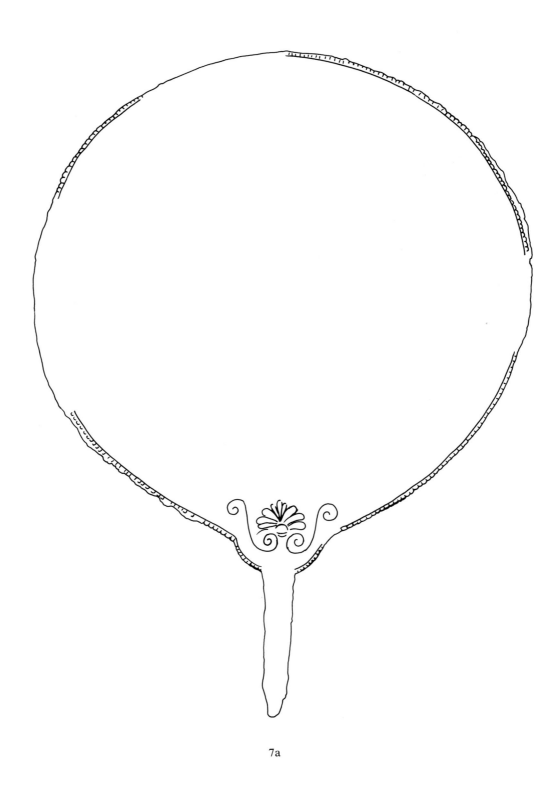

7a

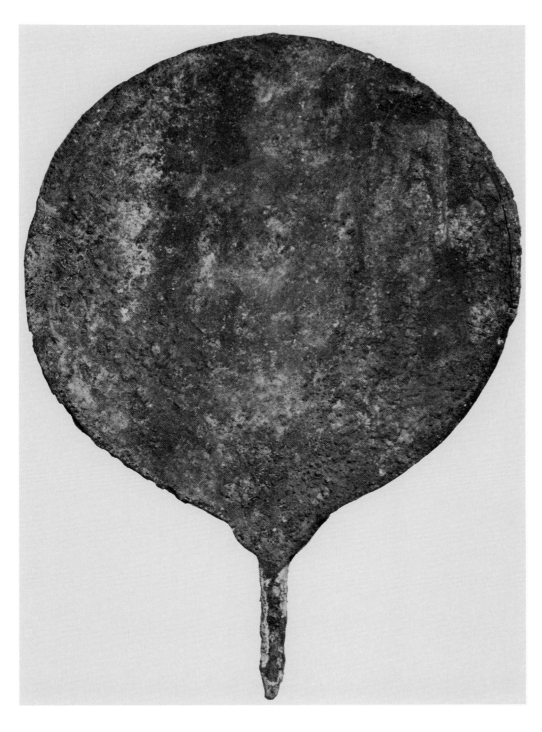

7b

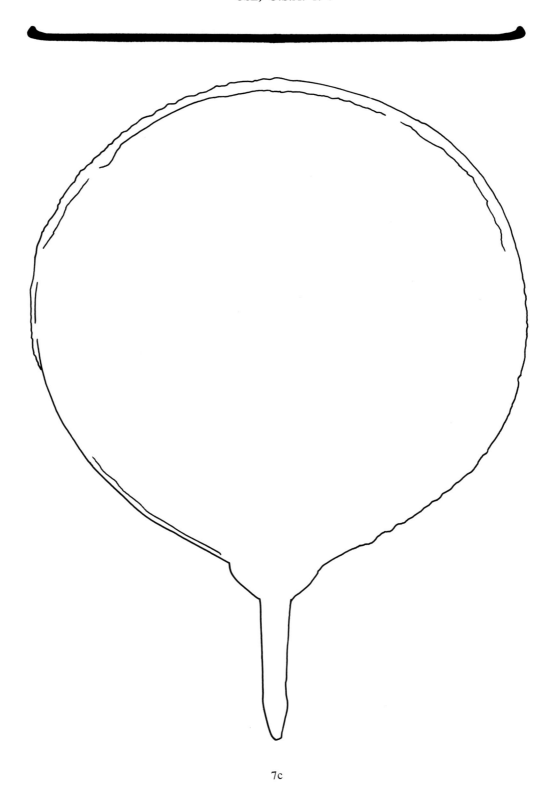

7c

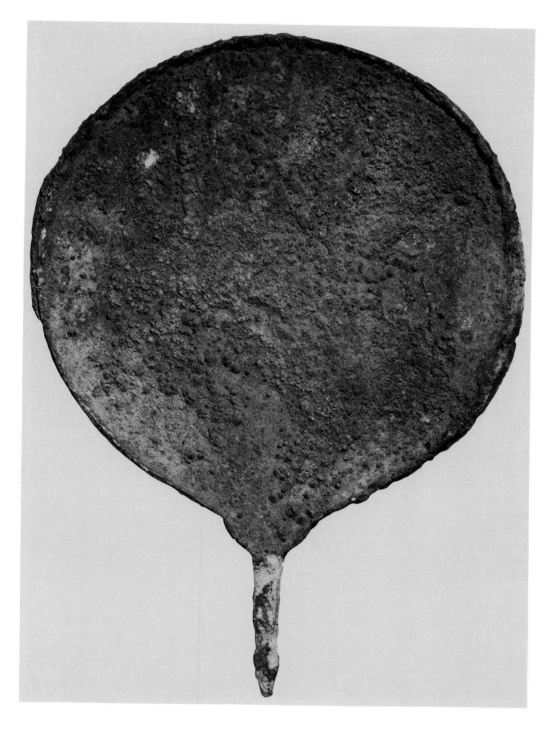

7d

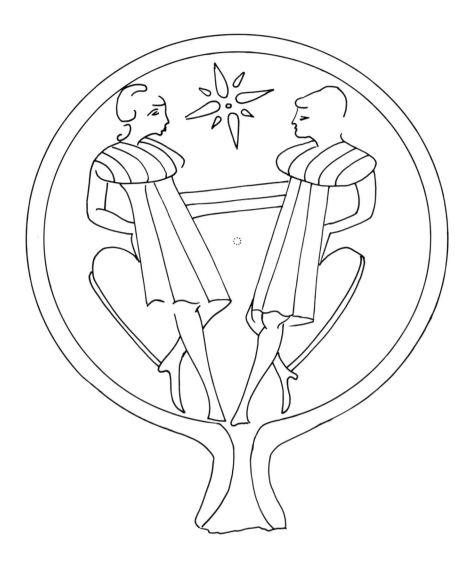

8a

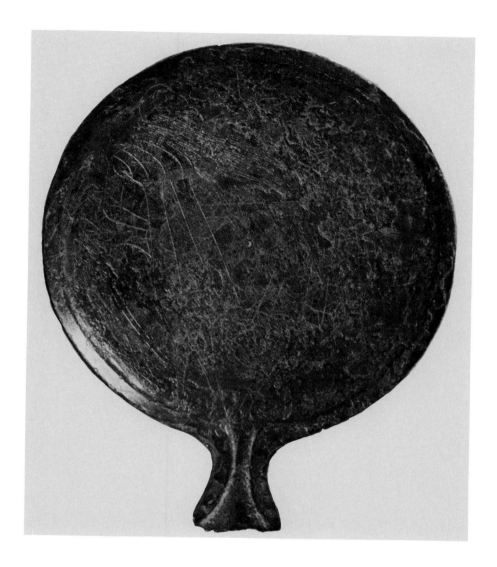

8b

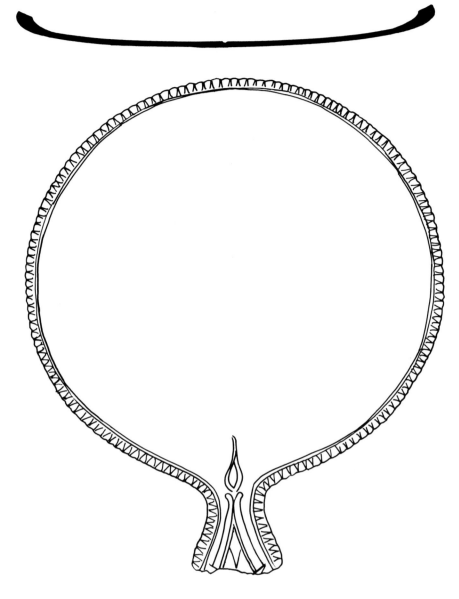

8c

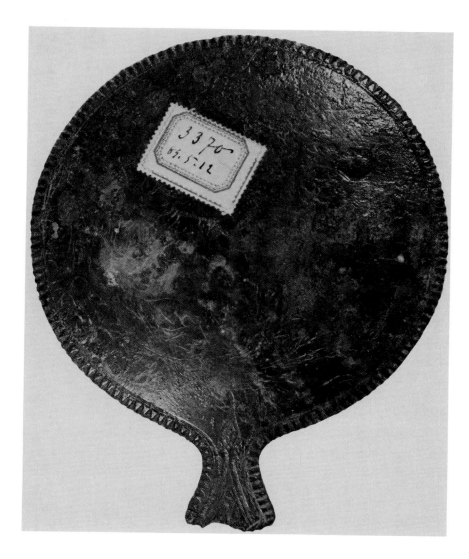

8d

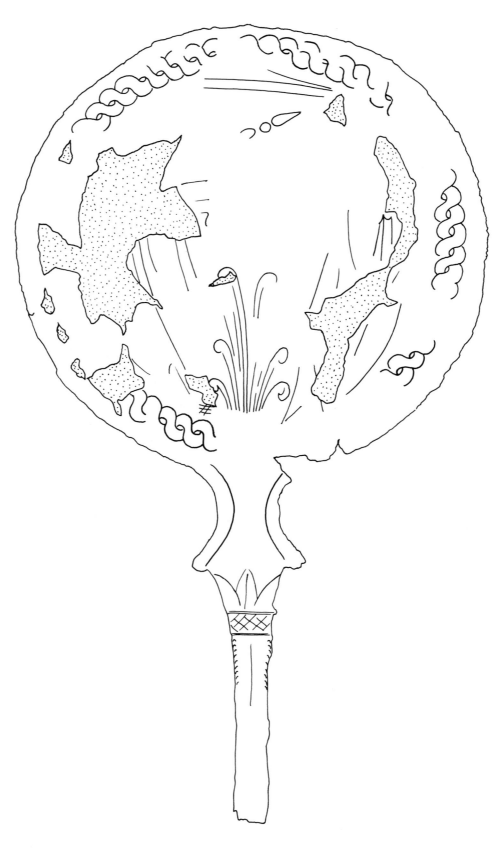

9a

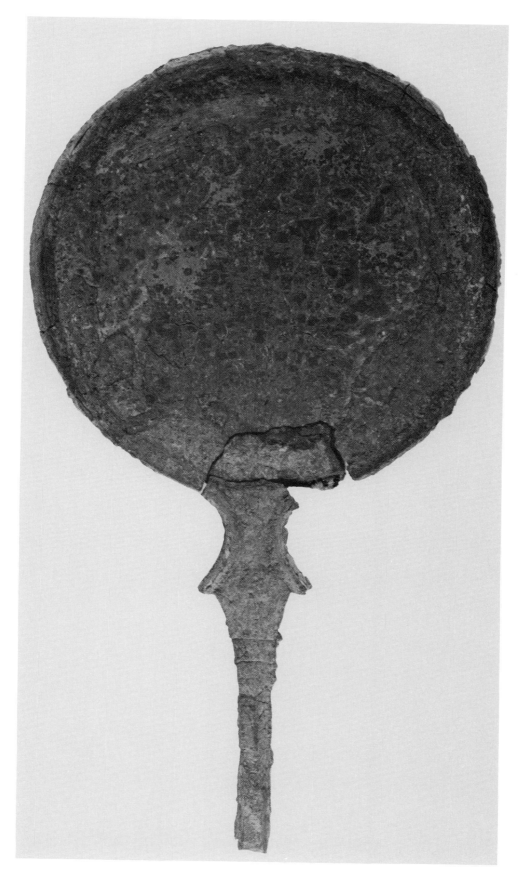

9b

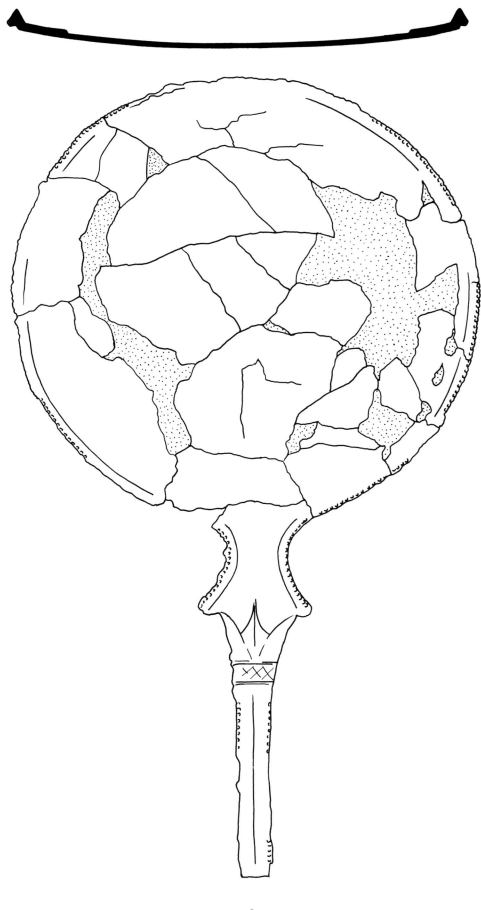

9c

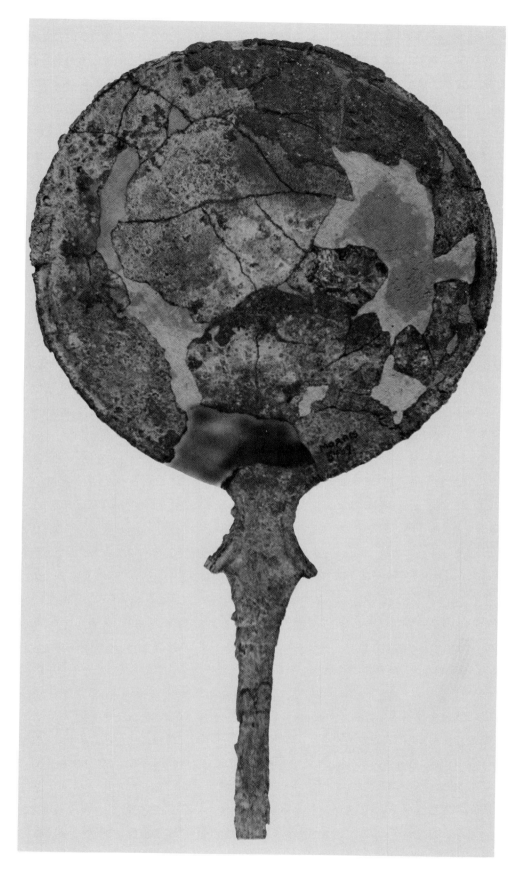

9d. 1: 9

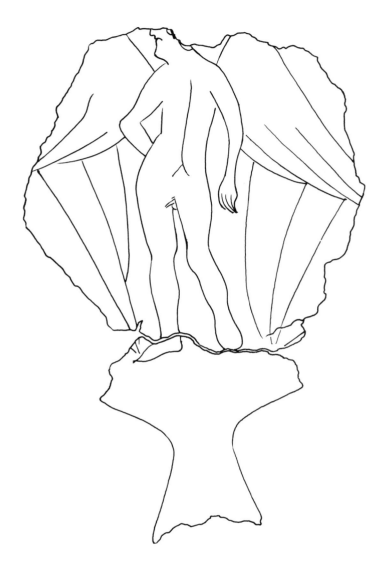

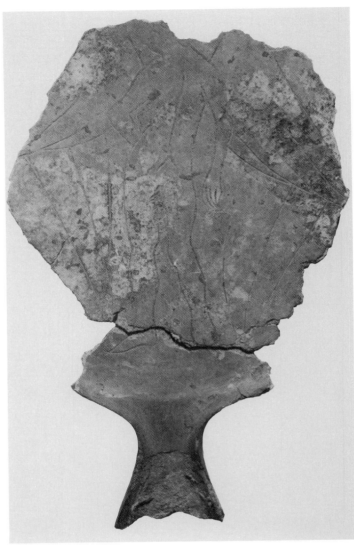

10a   10b

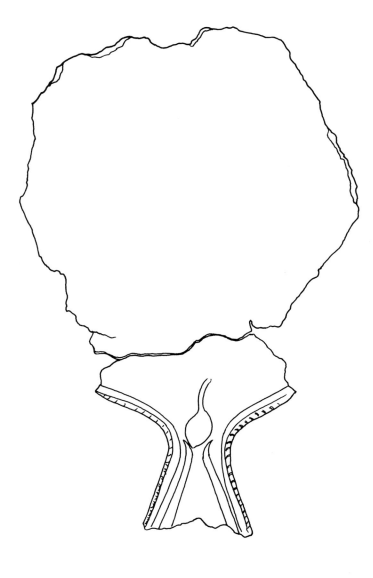

10c

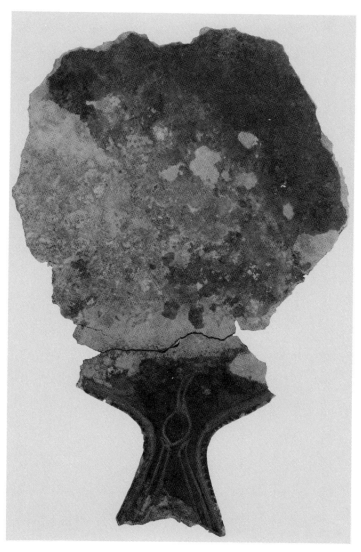

10d

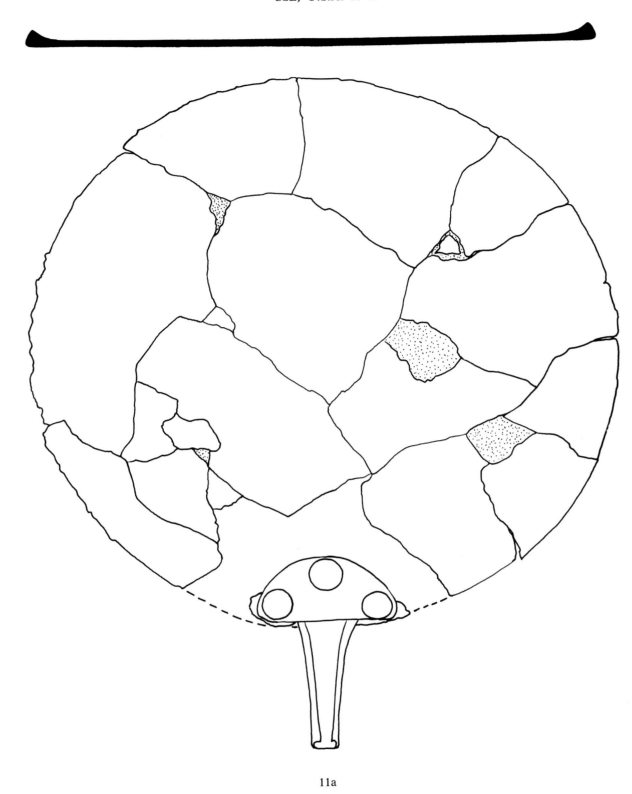

11a

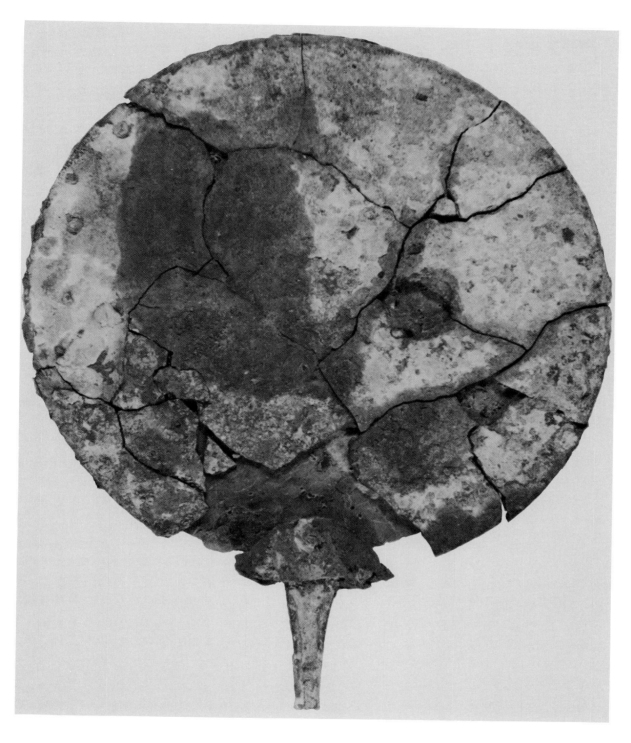

11b

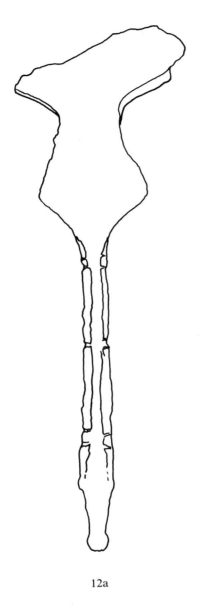

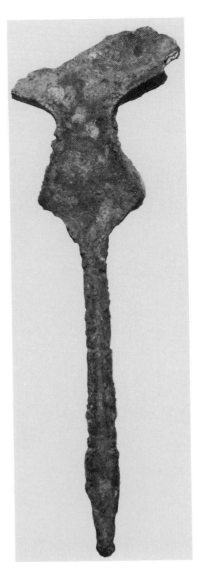

12a   12b

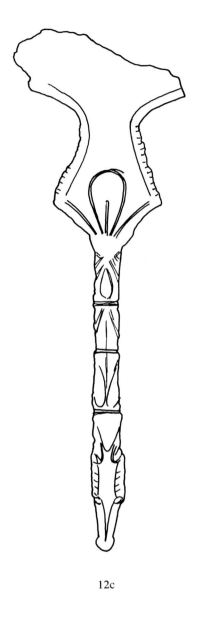

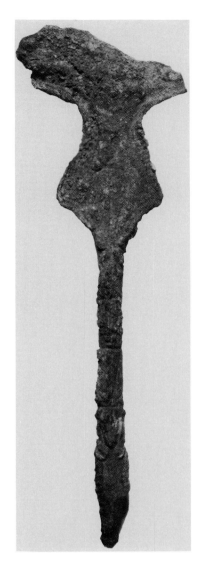

12c   12d

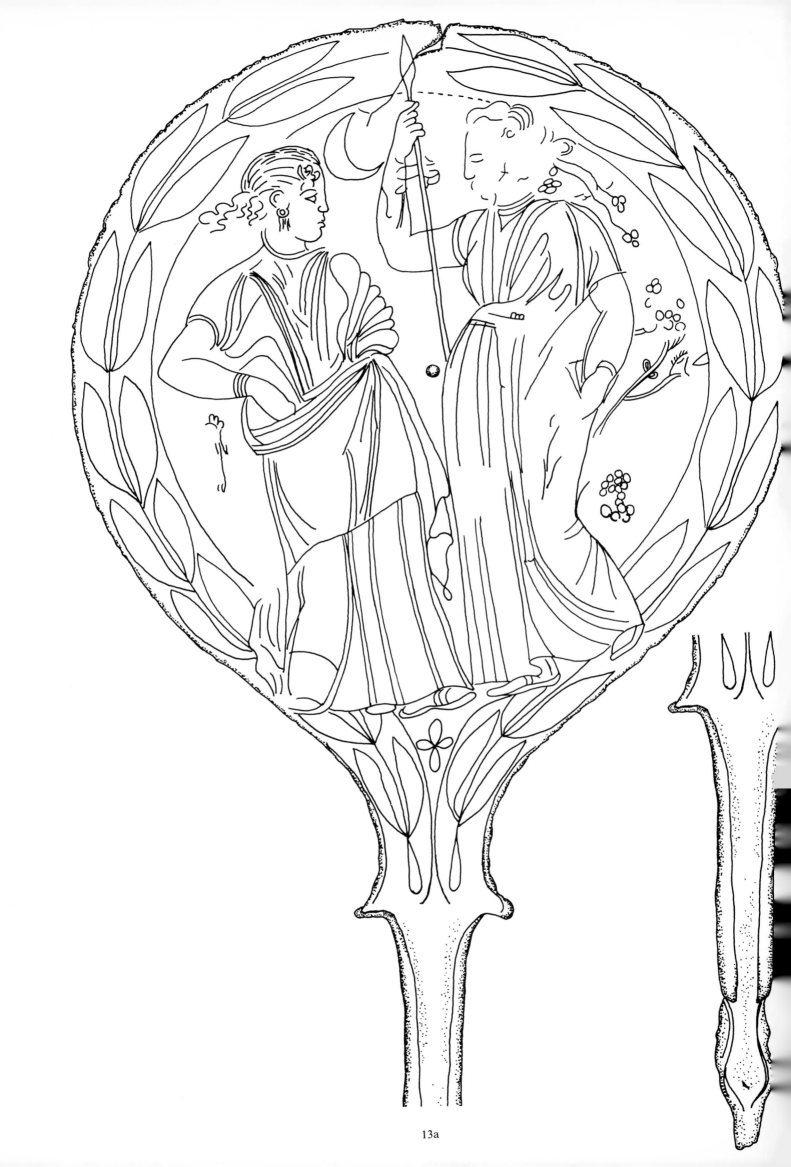

13a

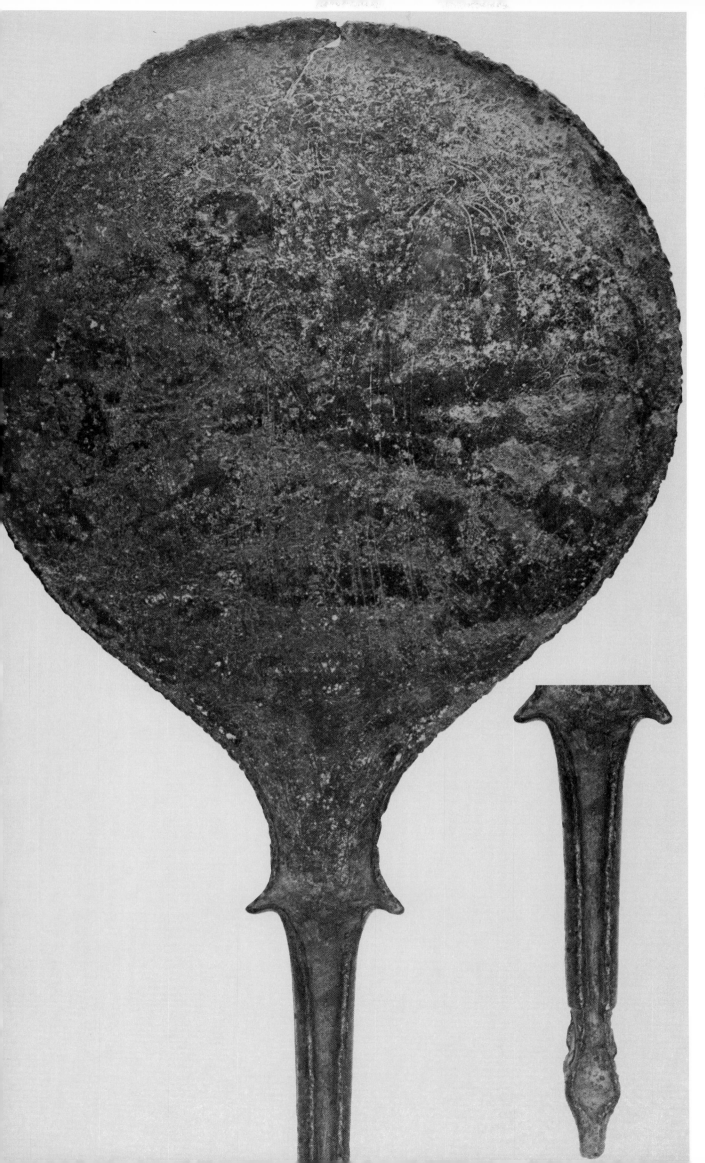

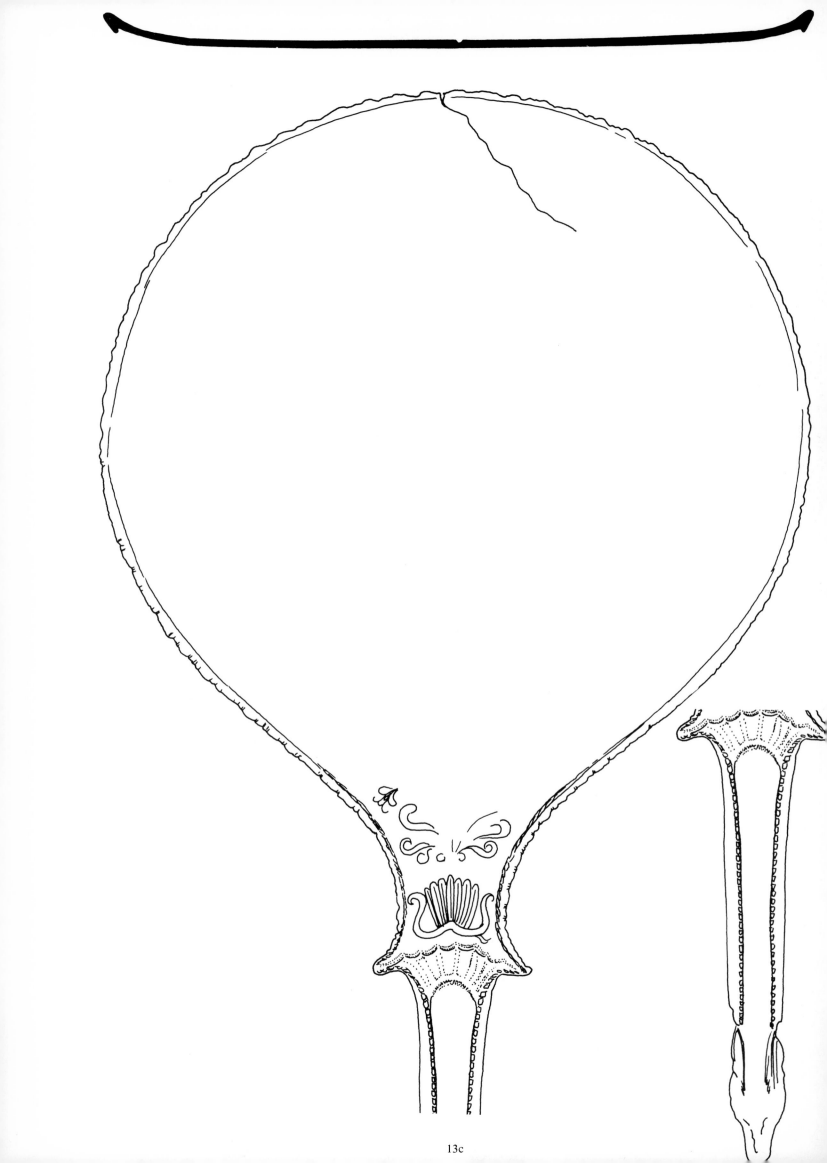

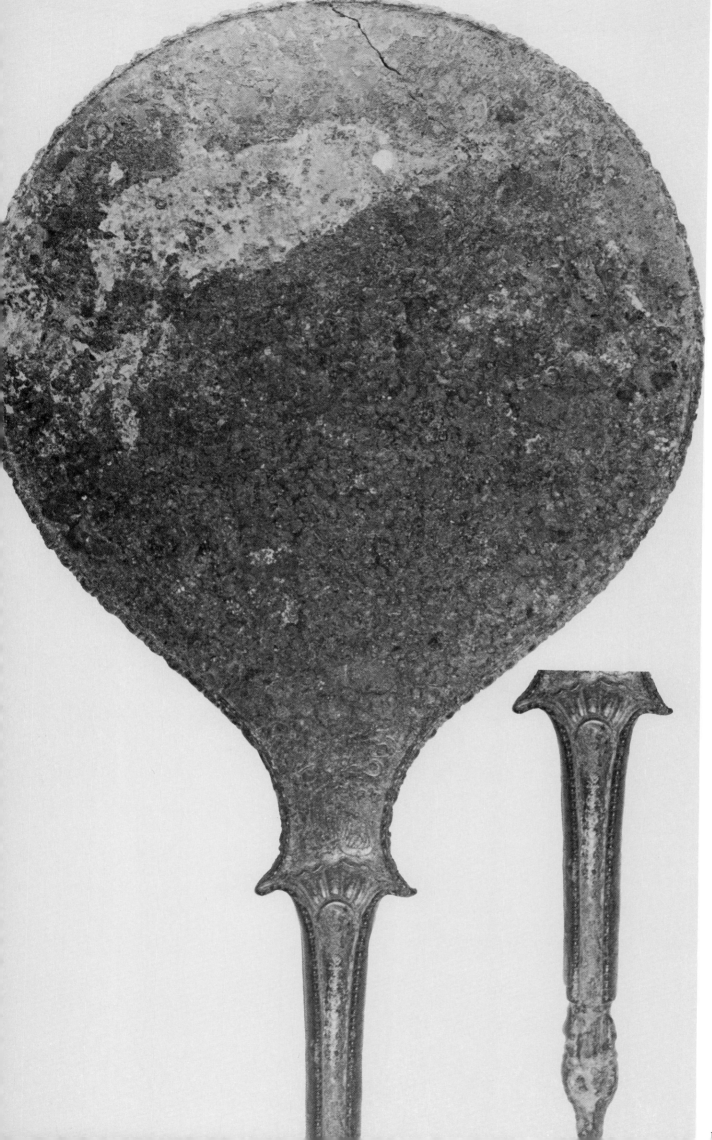

13d

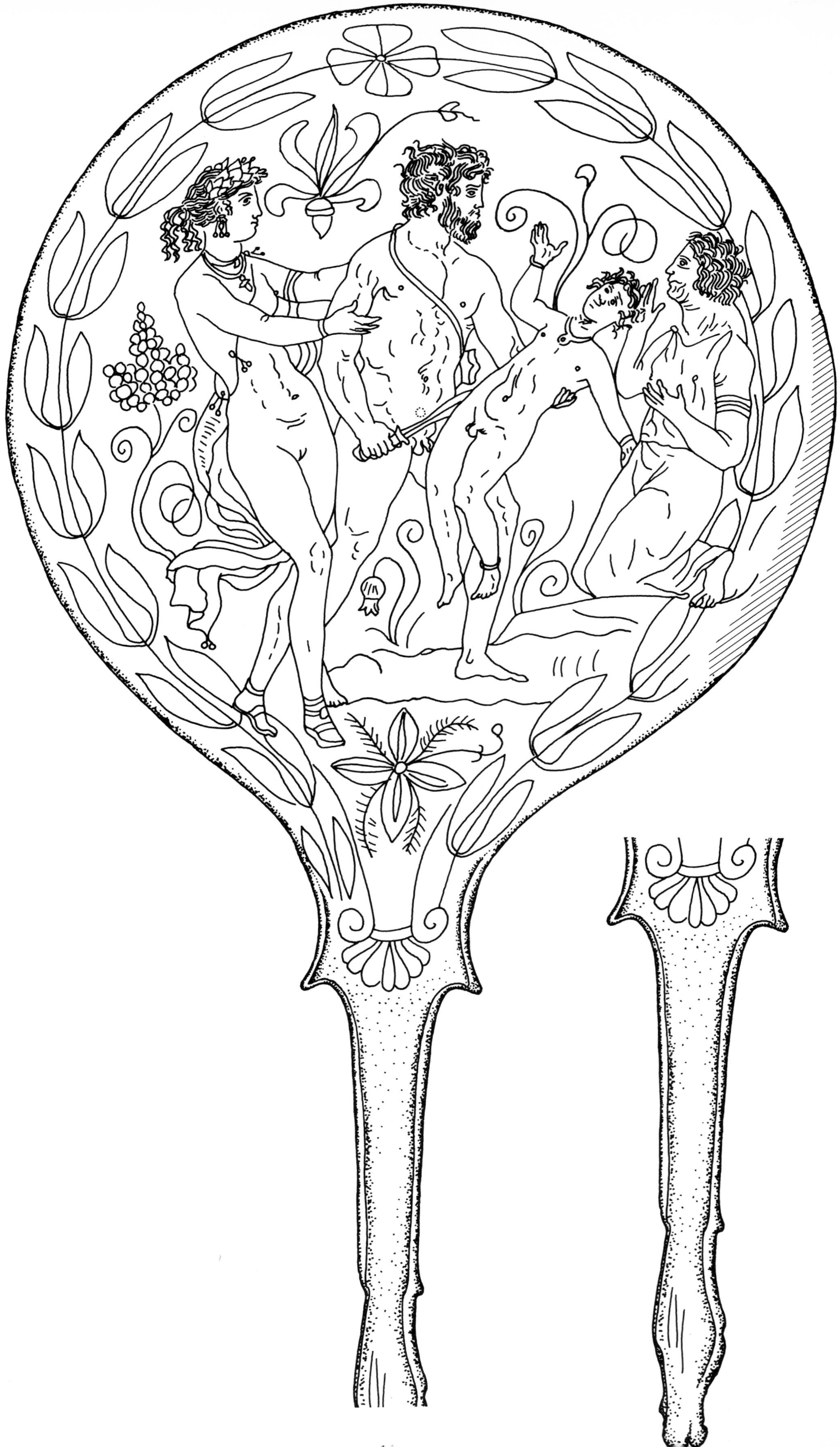

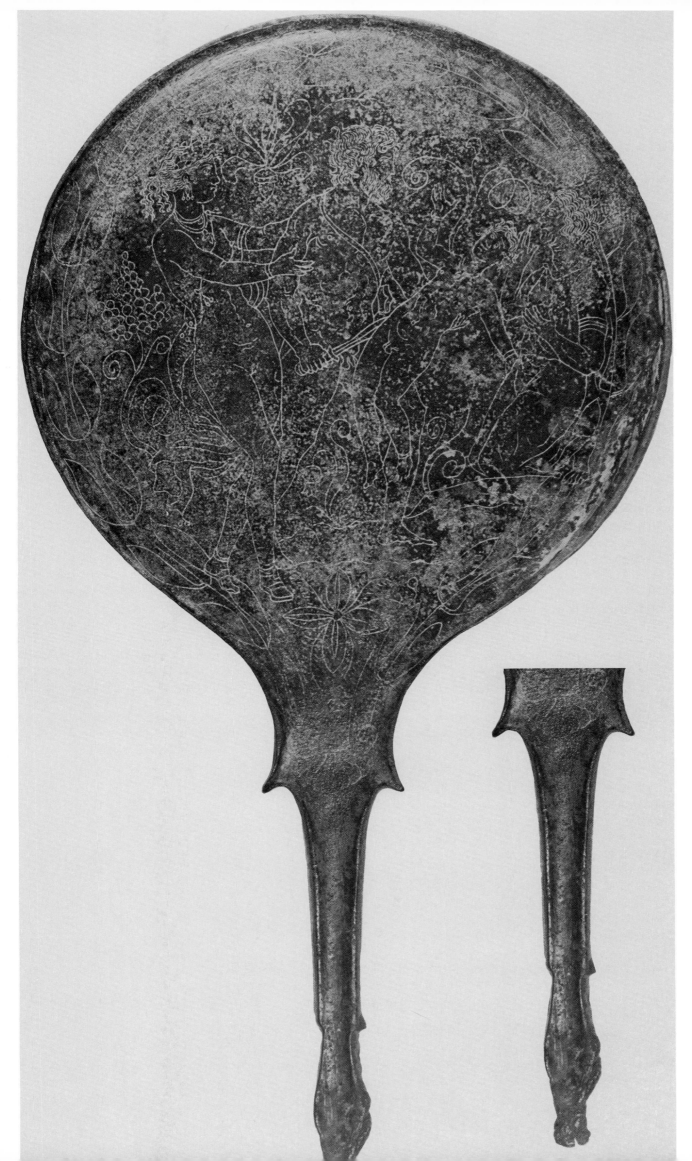

113

14b

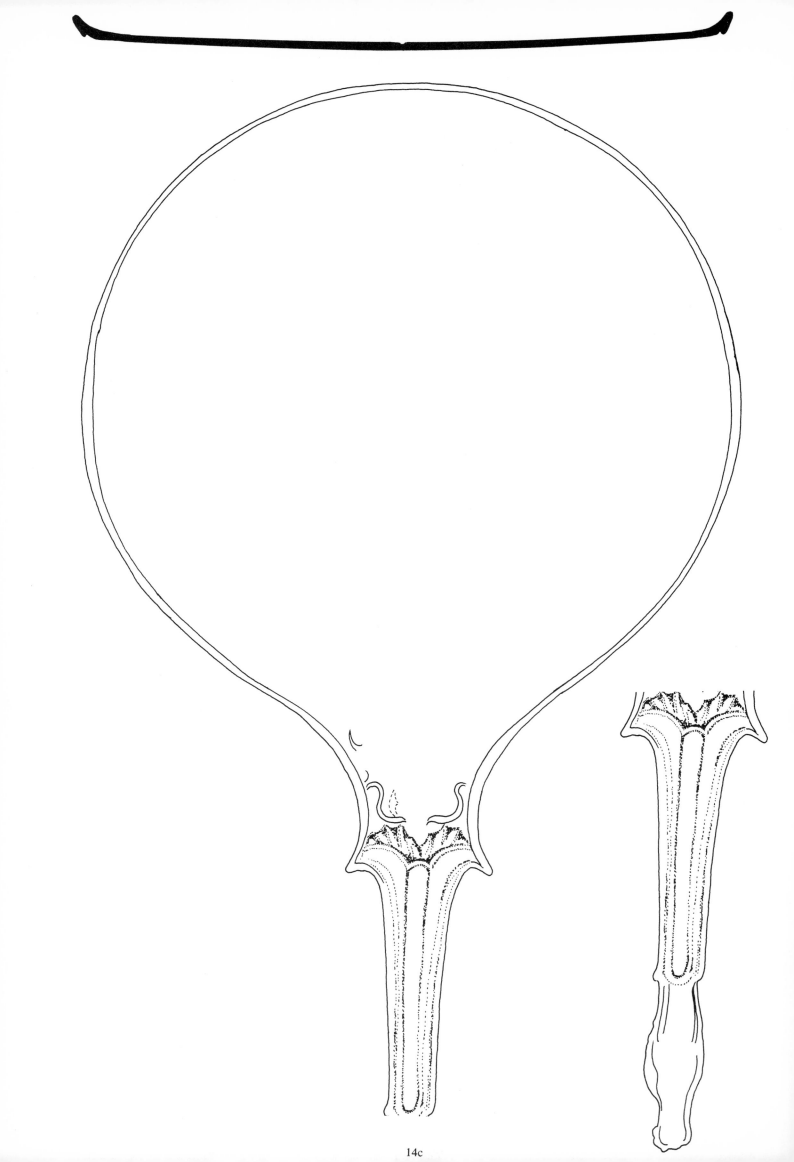

14c

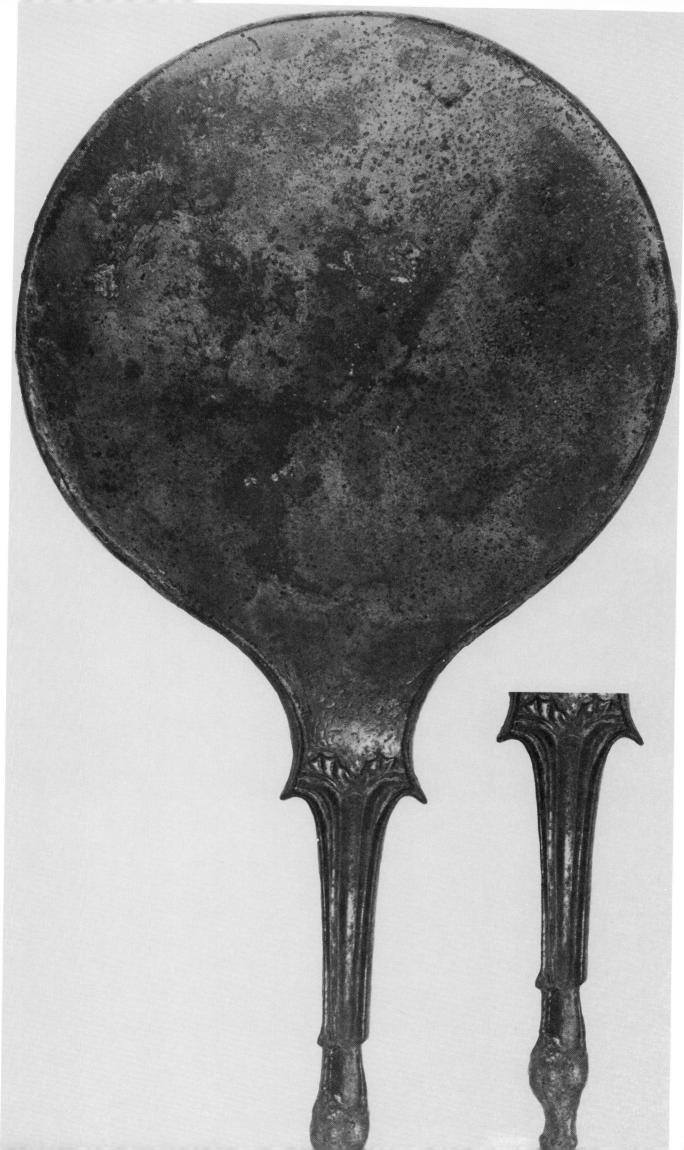

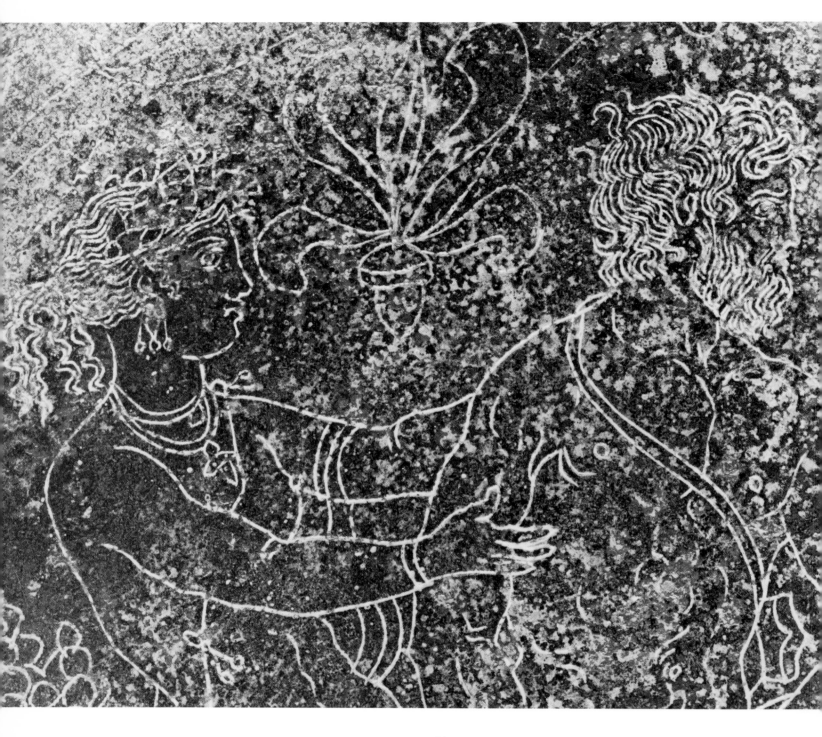

14e

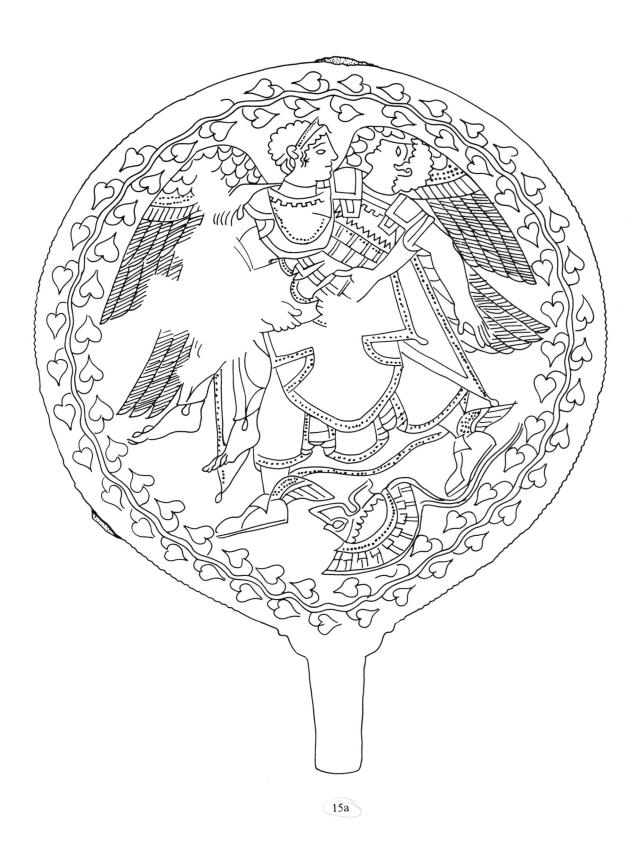

15a

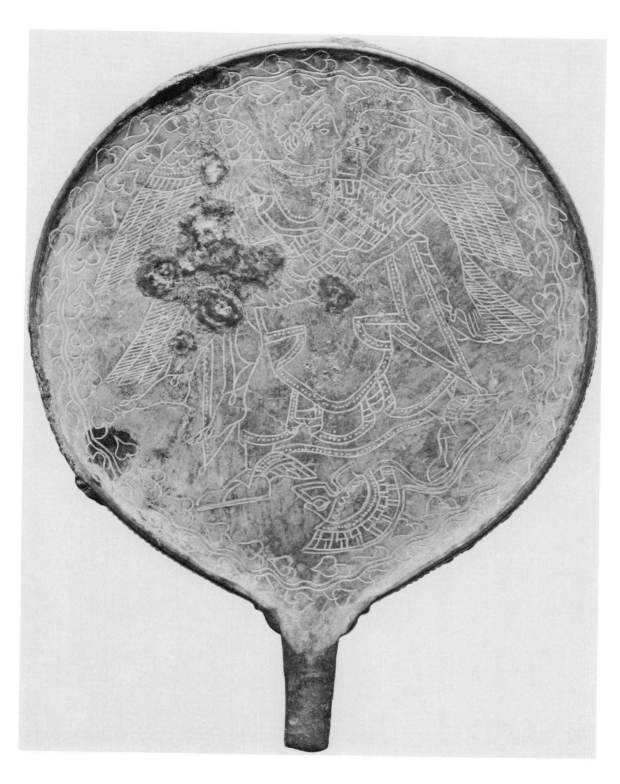

15b

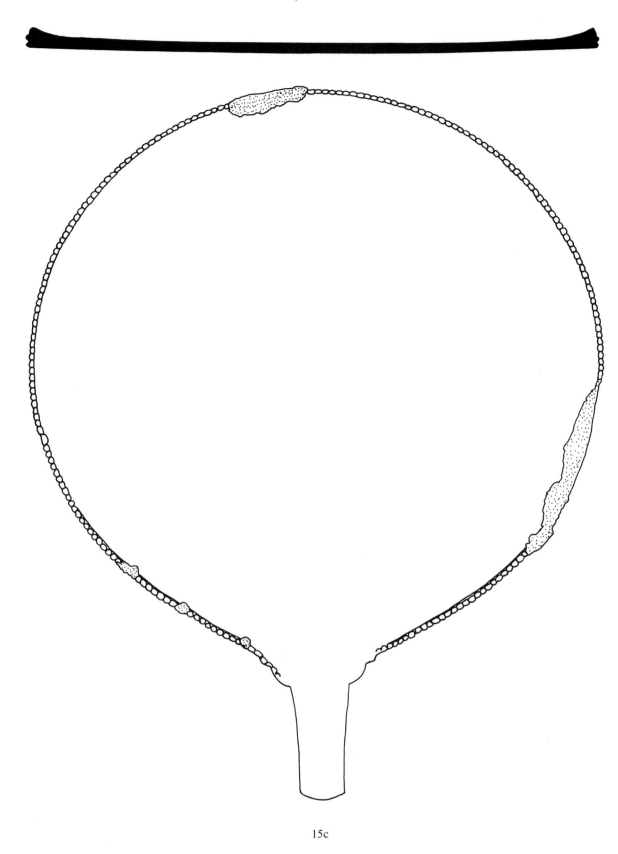

15c

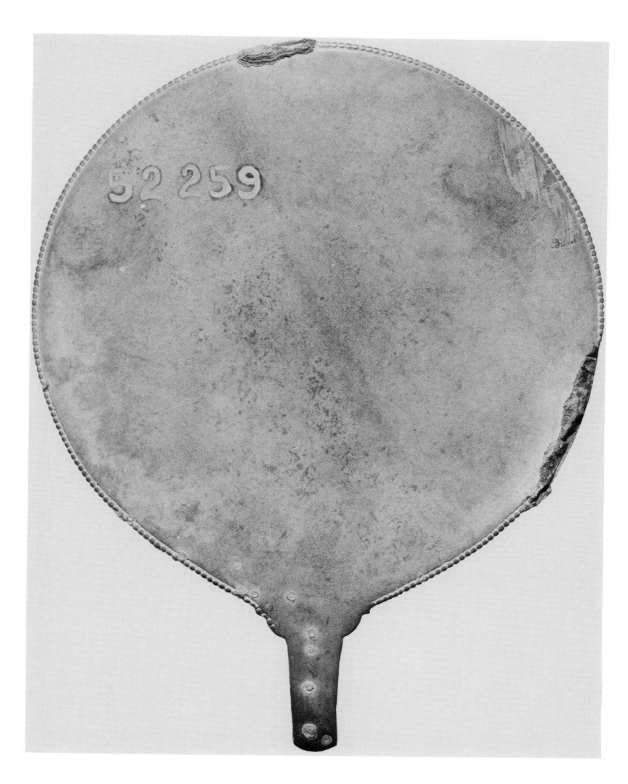

15d

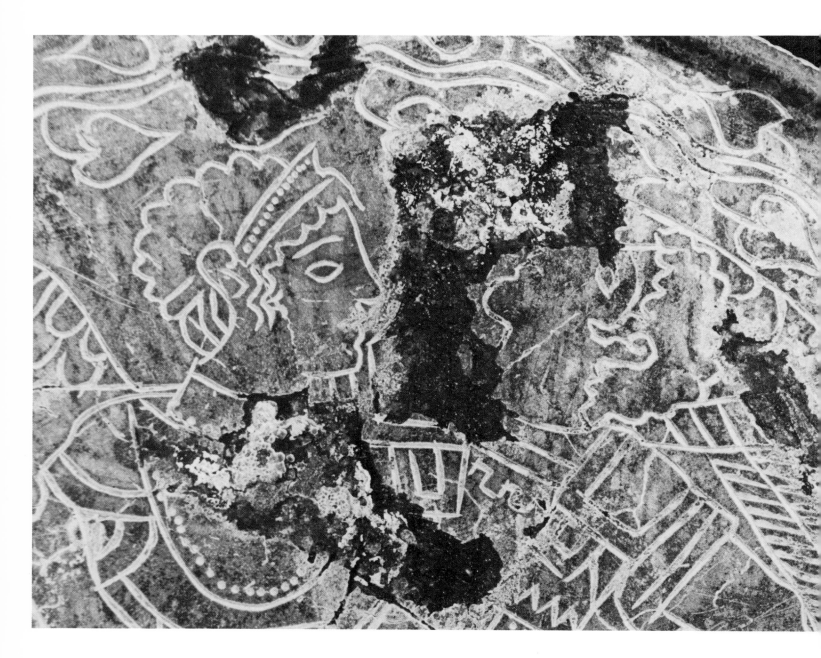

15e

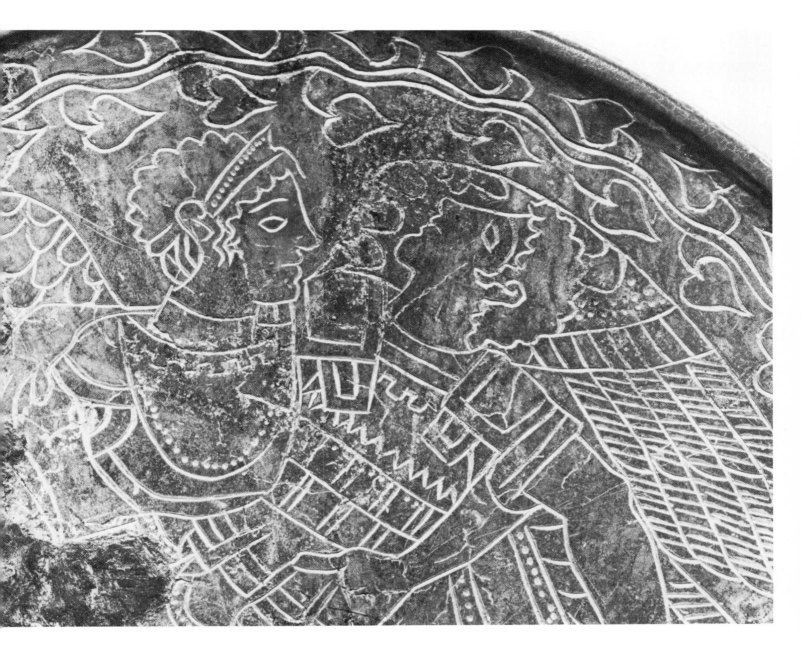

15f

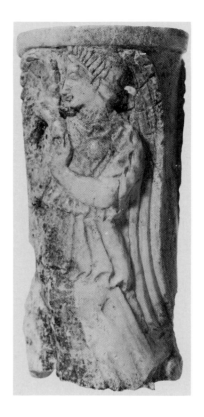

16a

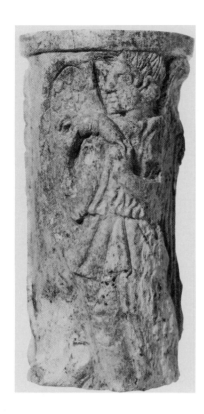

16b

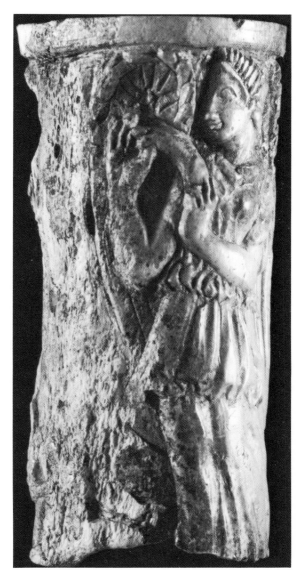

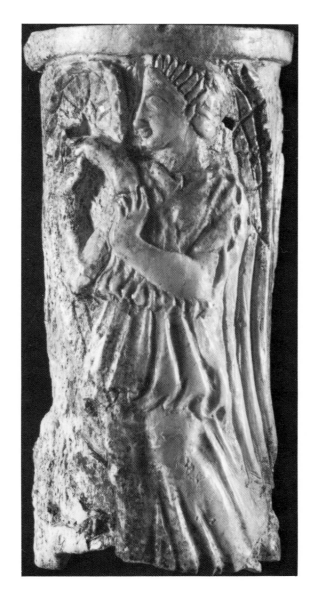

16c (*ca.* 1.5:1) 16d (*ca.* 1.5:1)

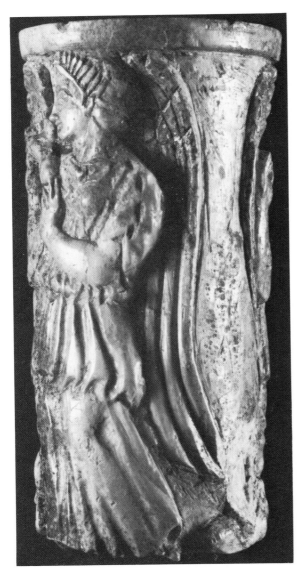

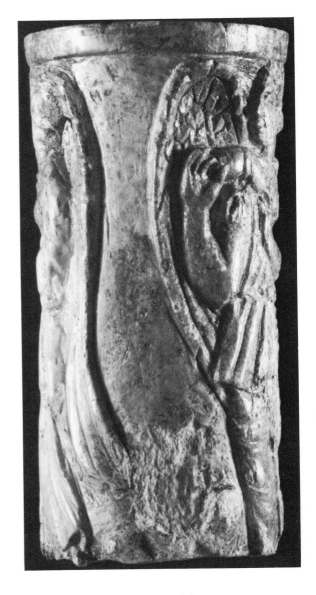

16e (*ca.* 1.5:1)   16f (*ca.* 1.5:1)

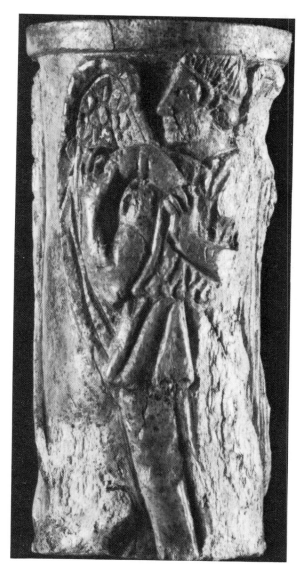

16g (*ca.* 1.5:1)

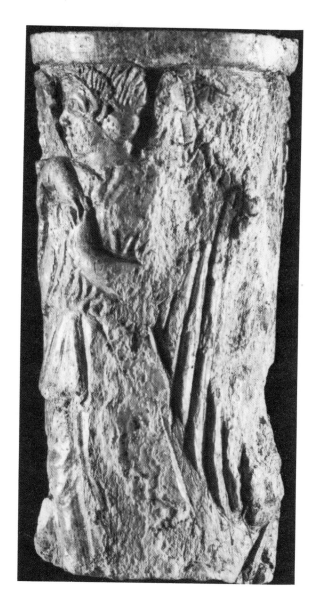

16h (*ca.* 1.5:1)

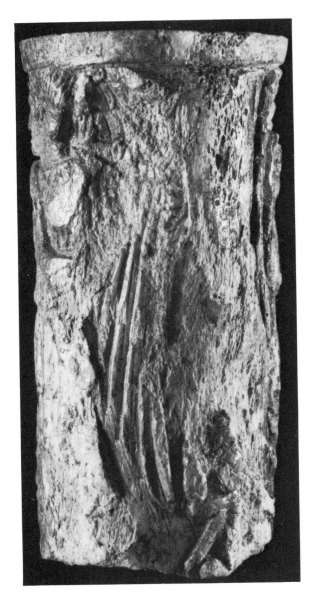

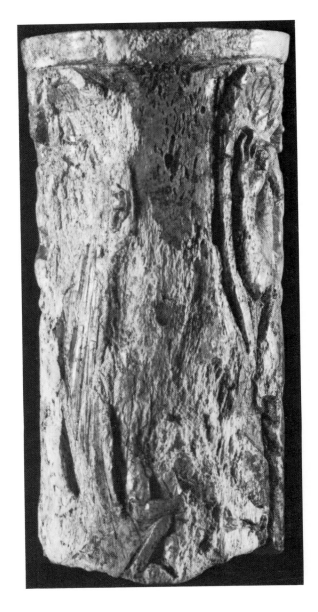

16i (*ca.* 1.5:1)   16j (*ca.* 1.5:1)

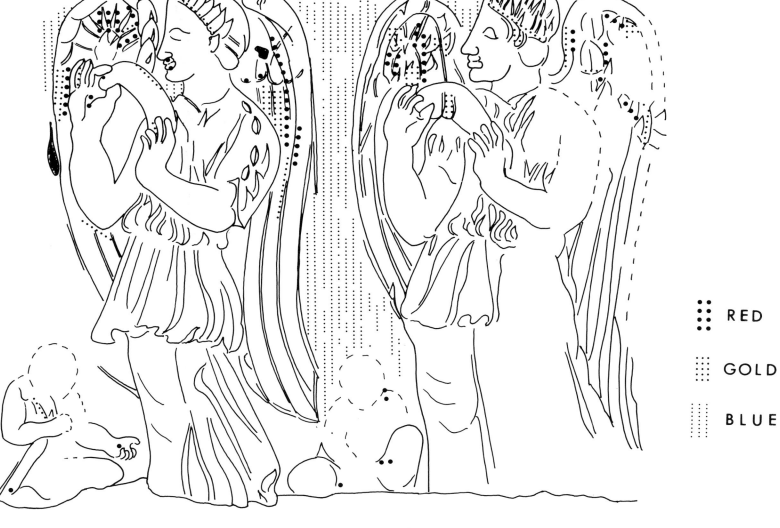

16k (*ca.* 1.5:1)

RED

GOLD

BLUE

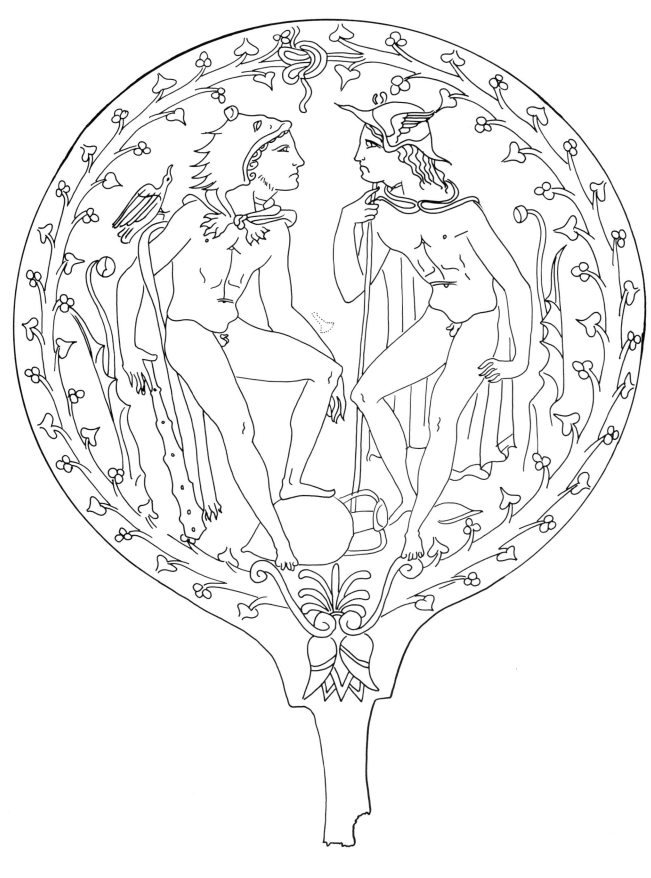

17a

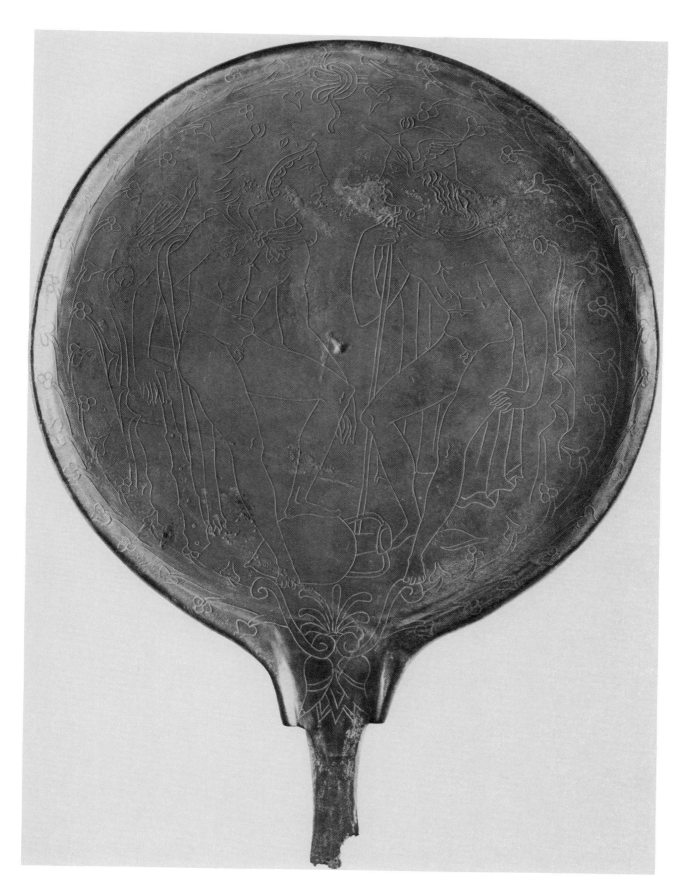

17b

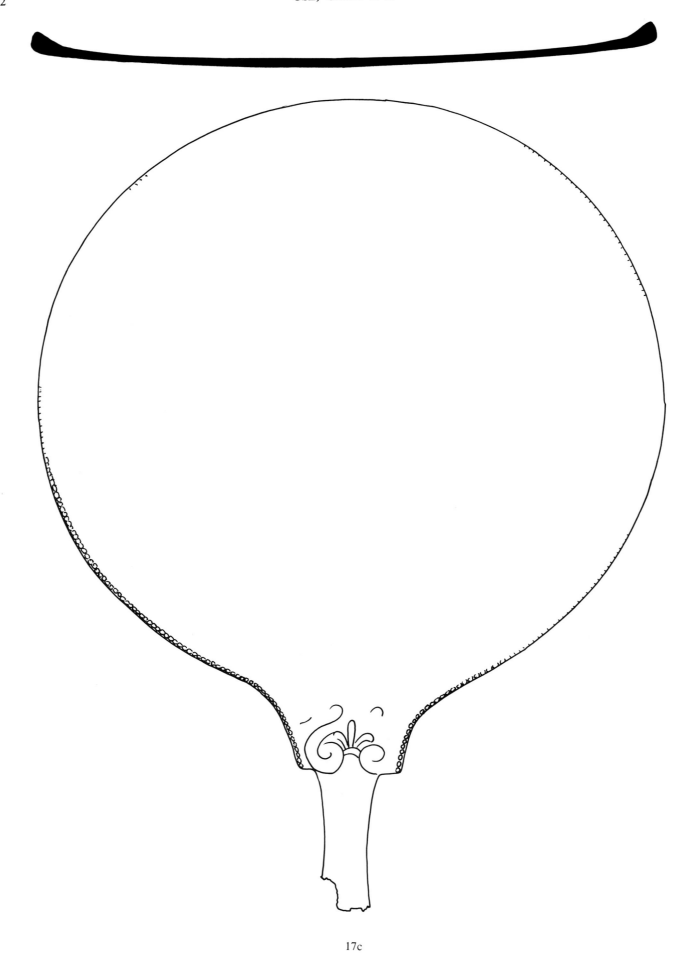

17c

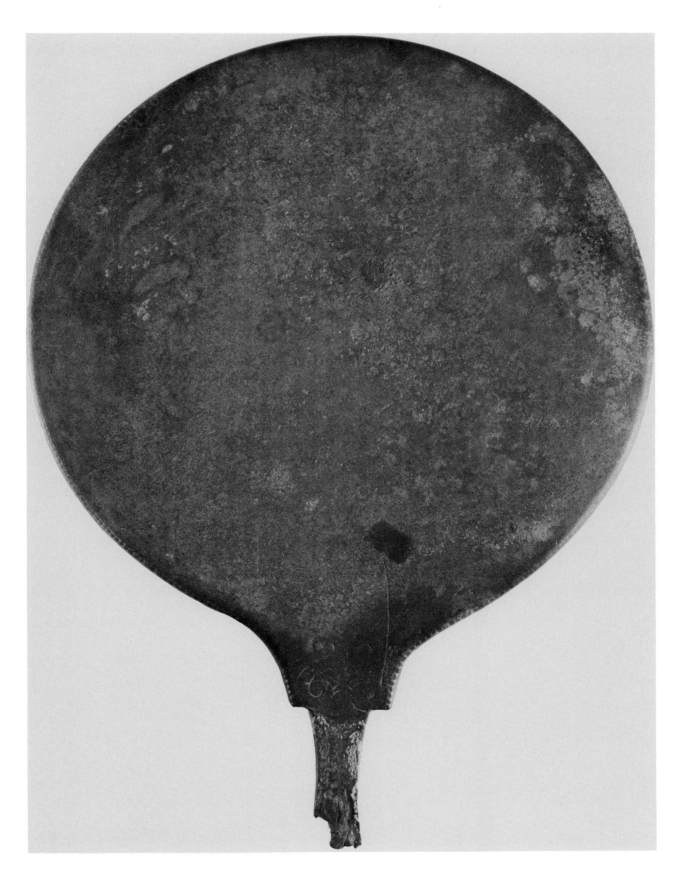

17d

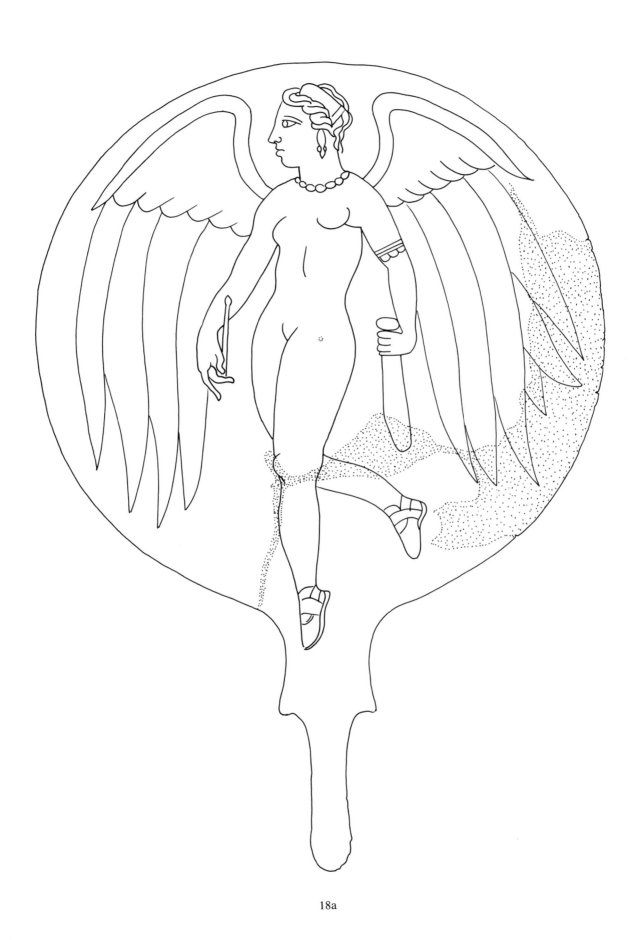

18a

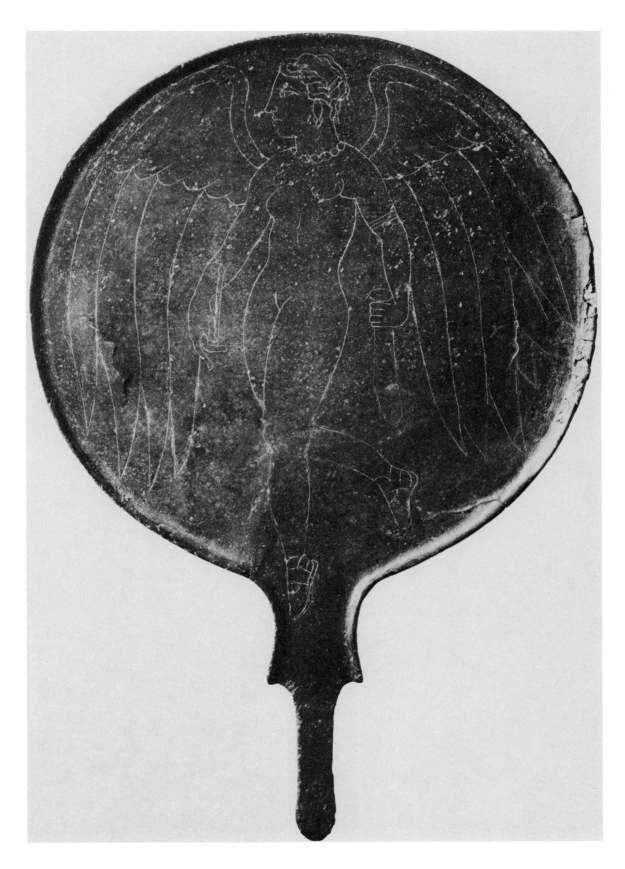

18b

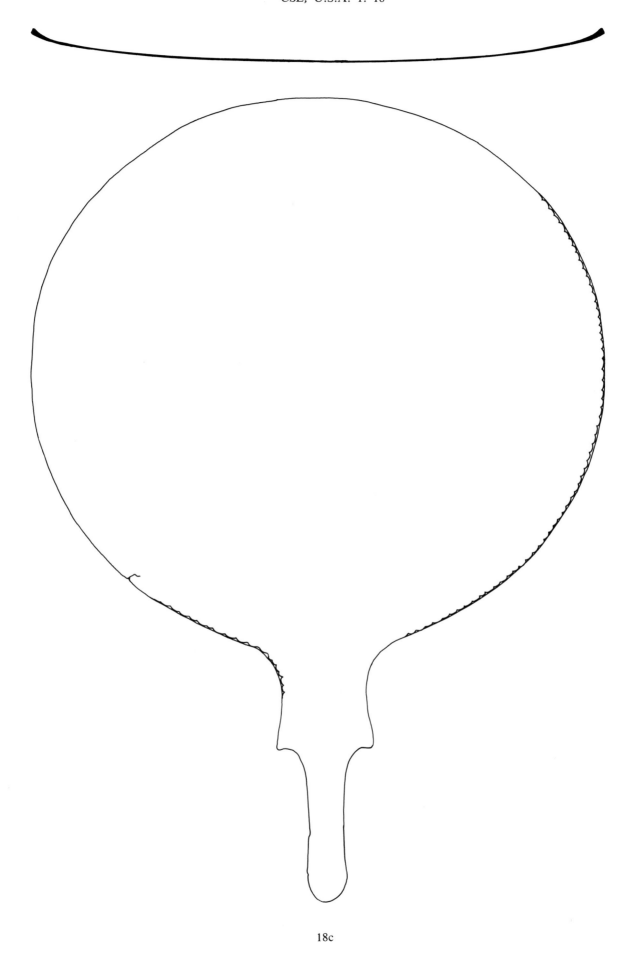

18c. 1: 18

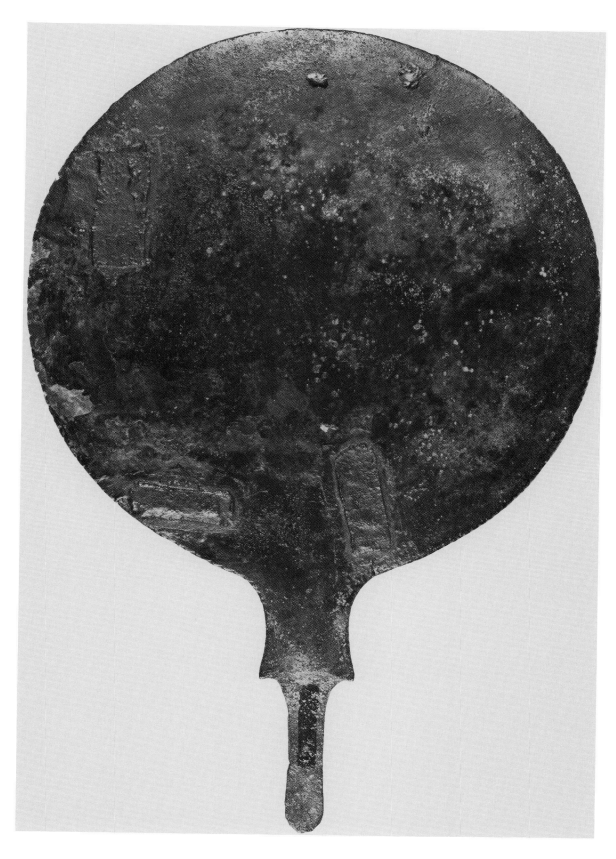

18d

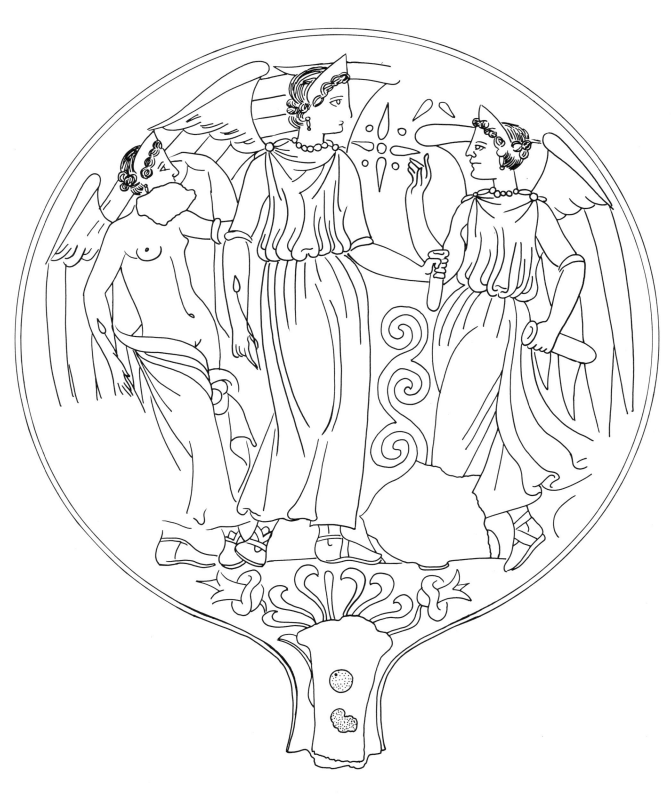

19a

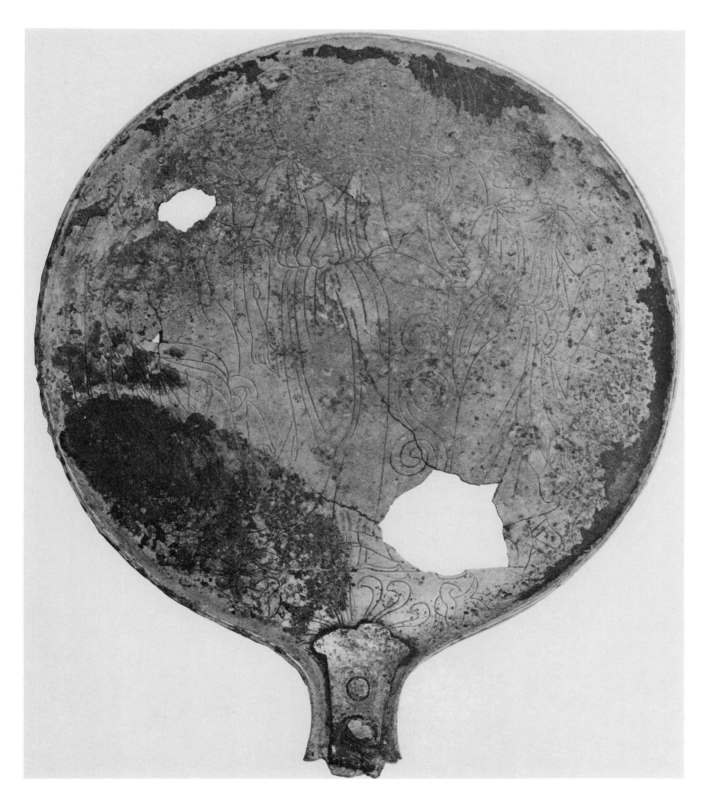

19b

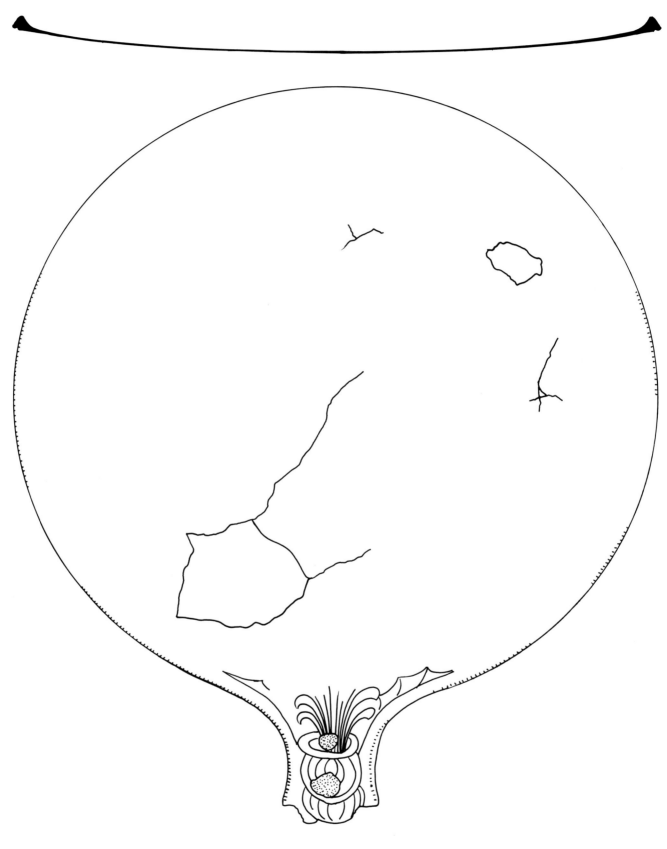

19c

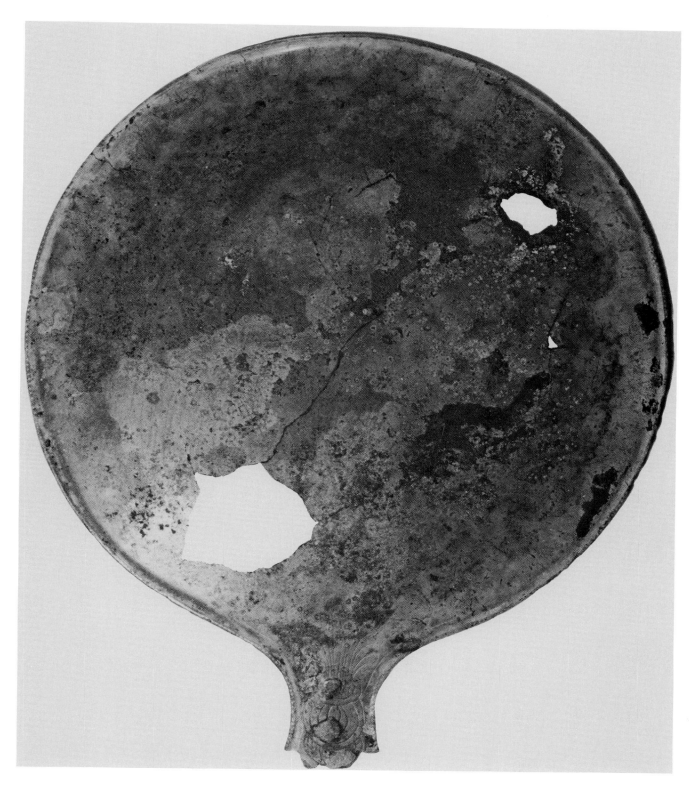

19d

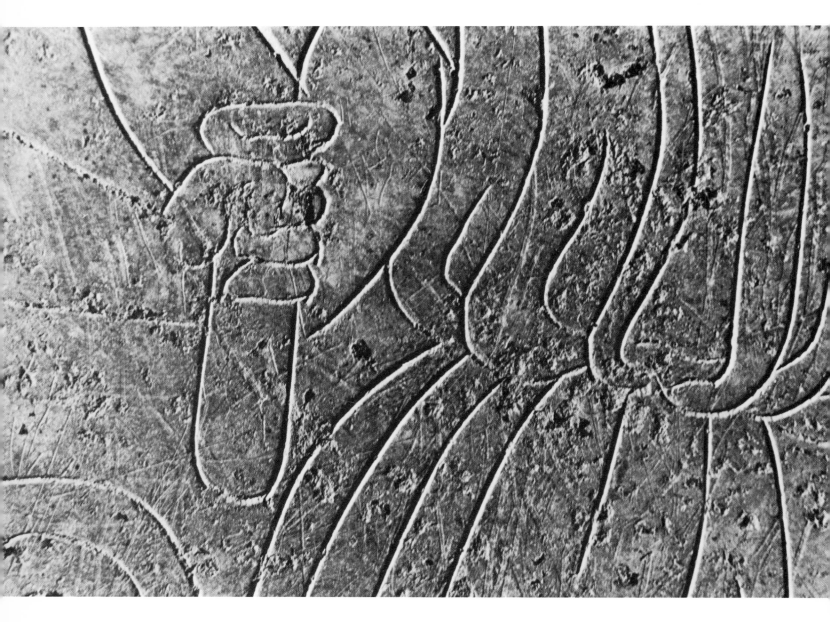

19e

144

20a

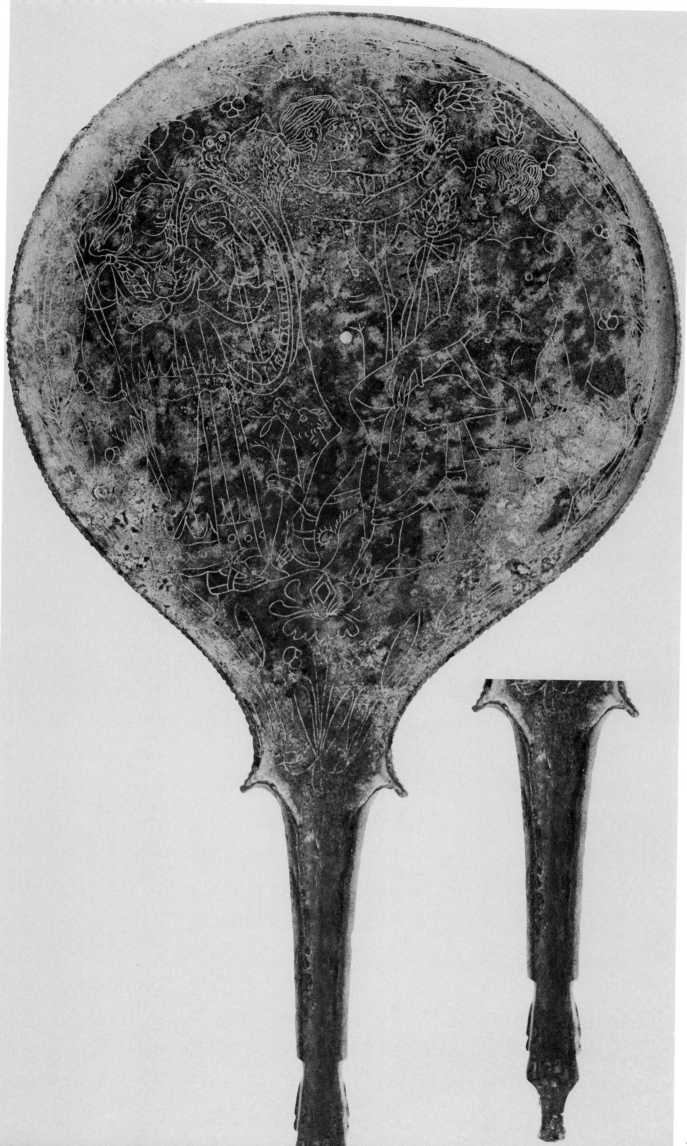

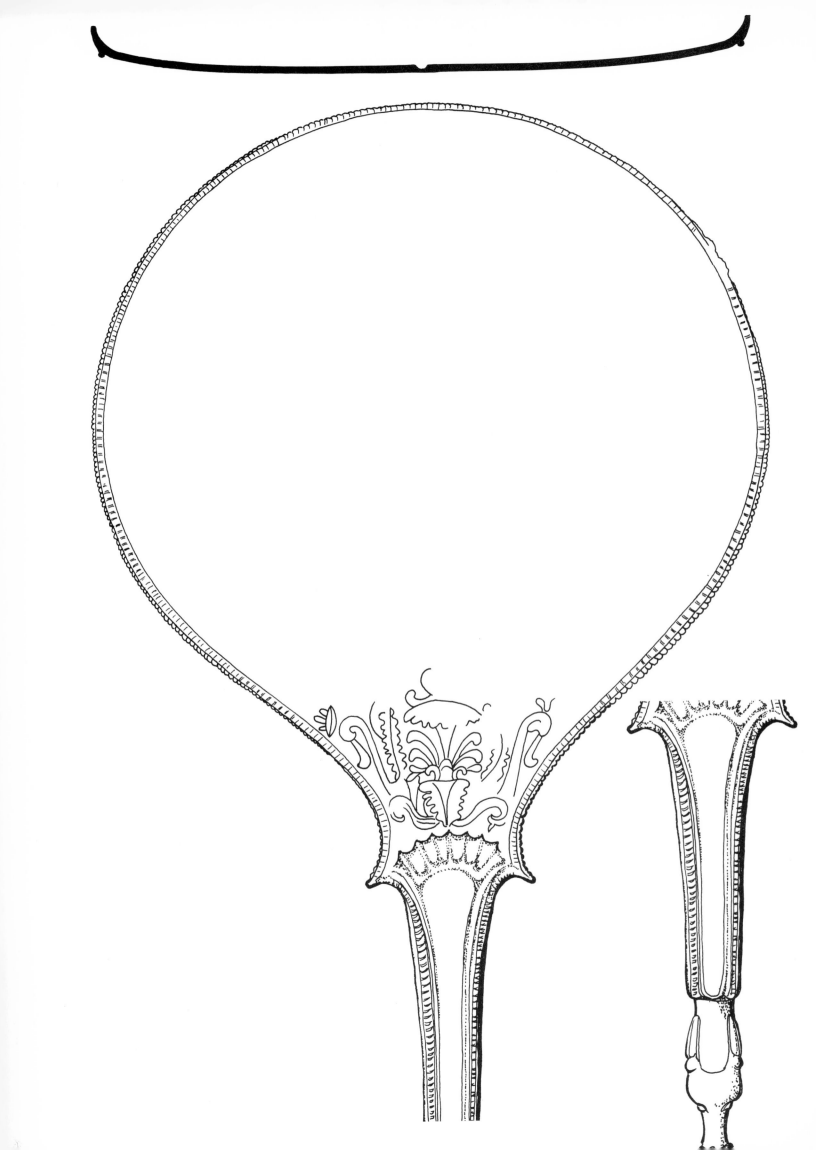

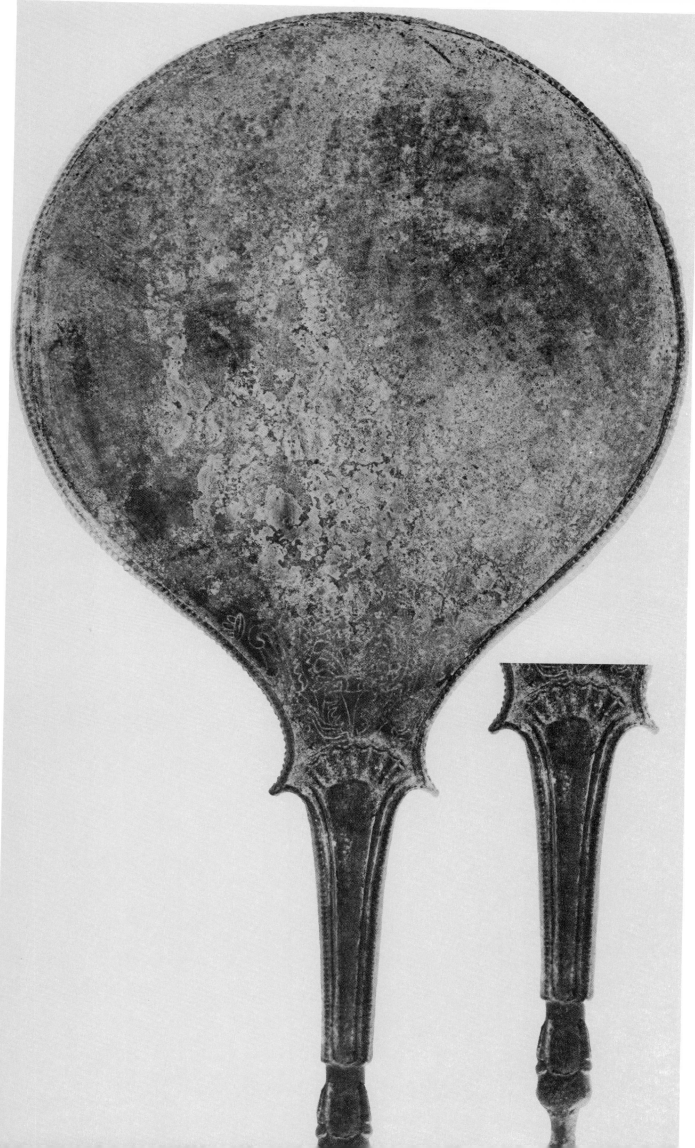

148

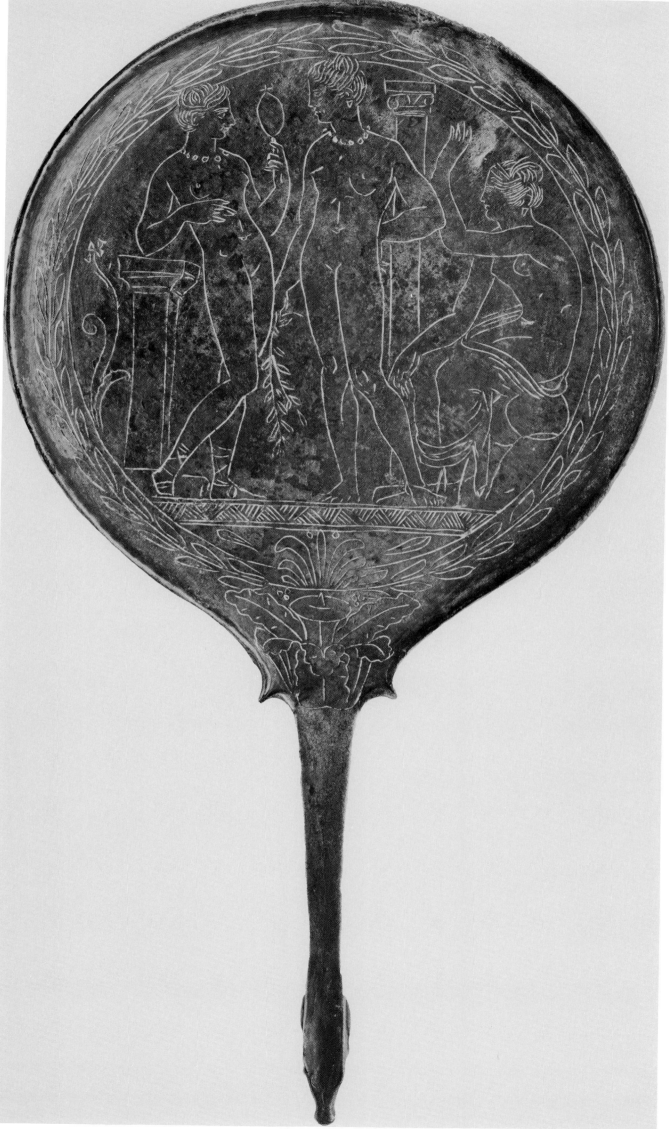

150

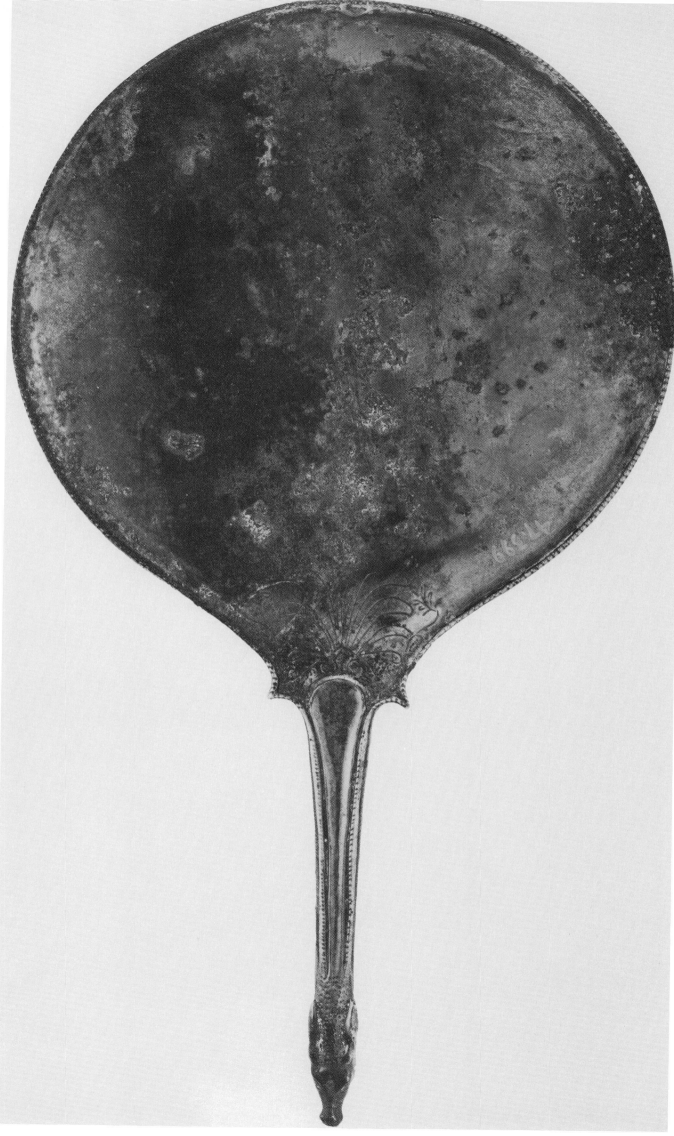

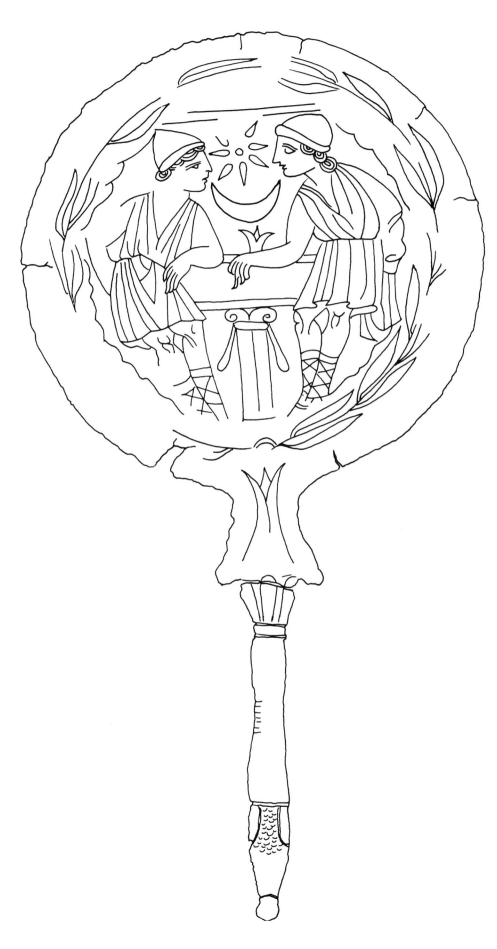

22a

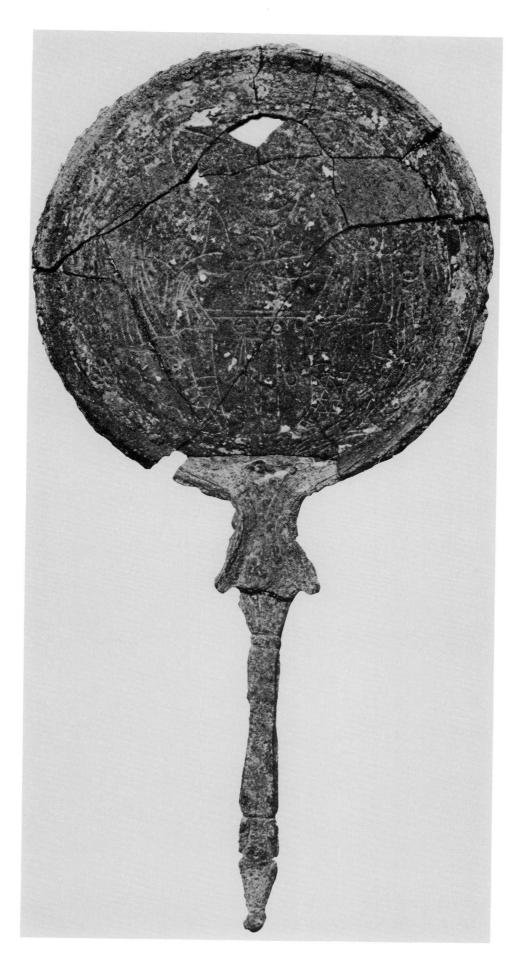

22b

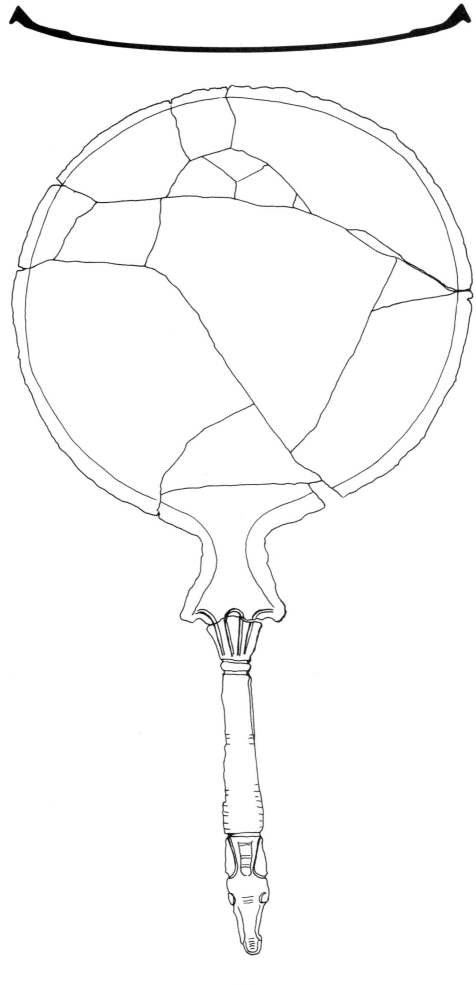

22c

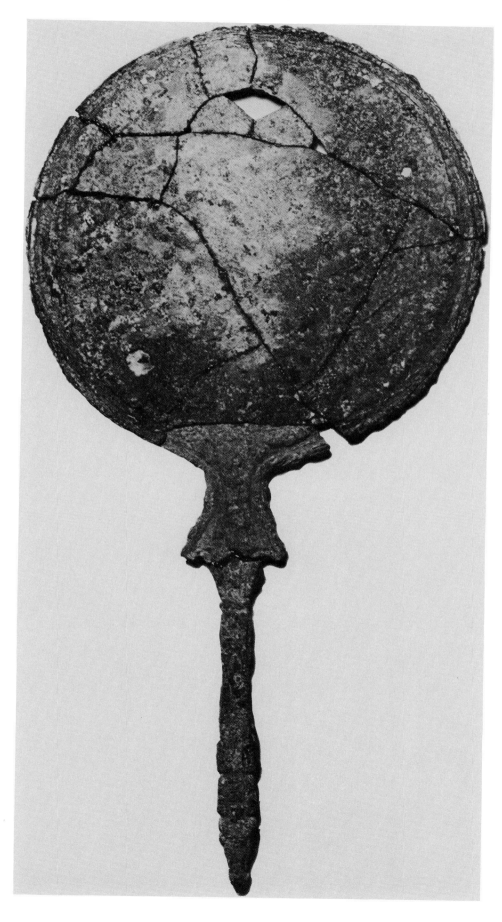

22d

156

23a

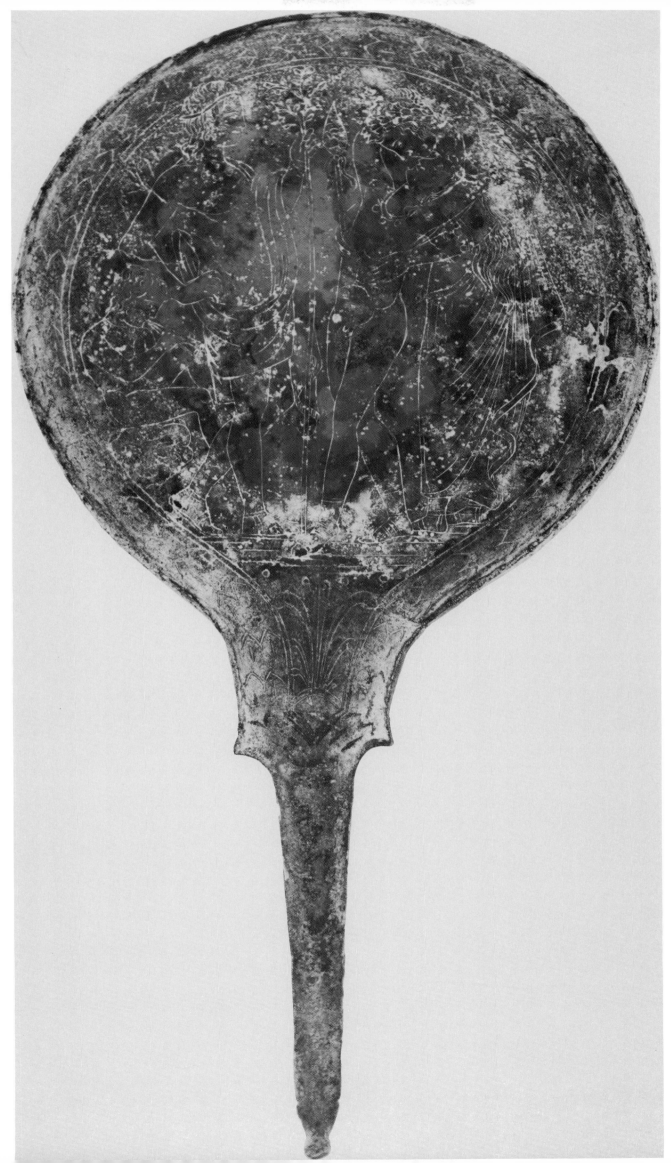

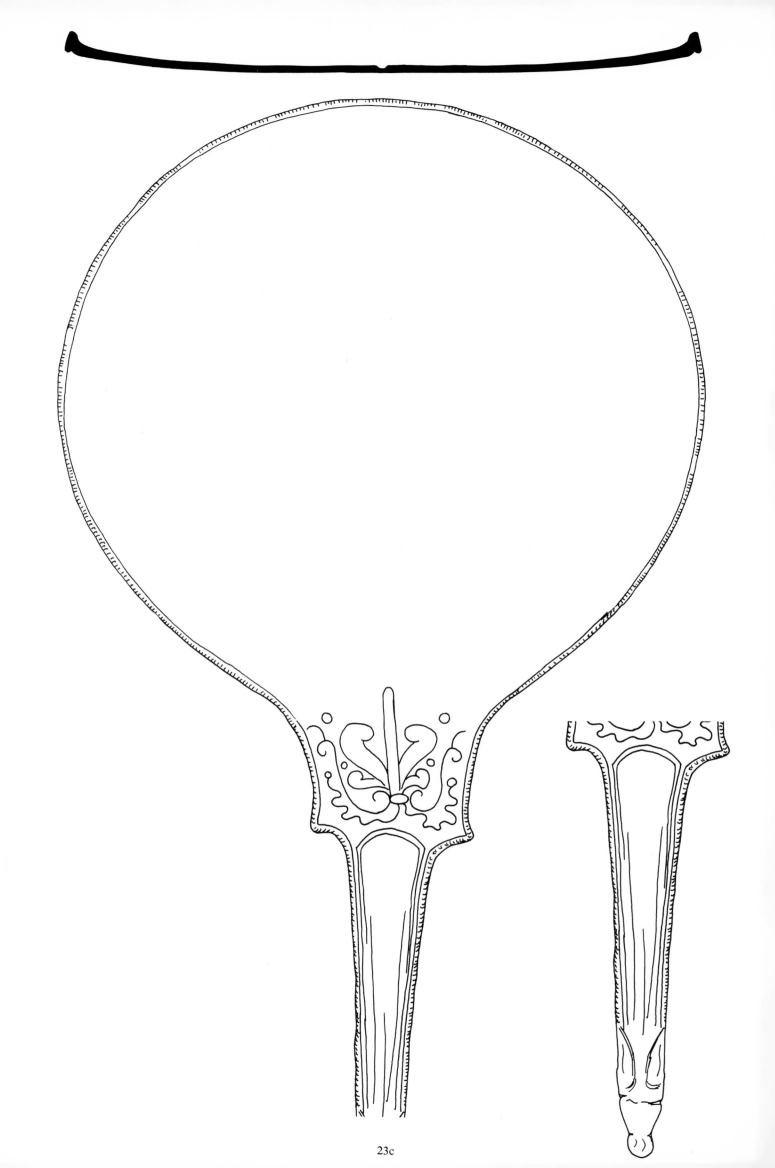

23c

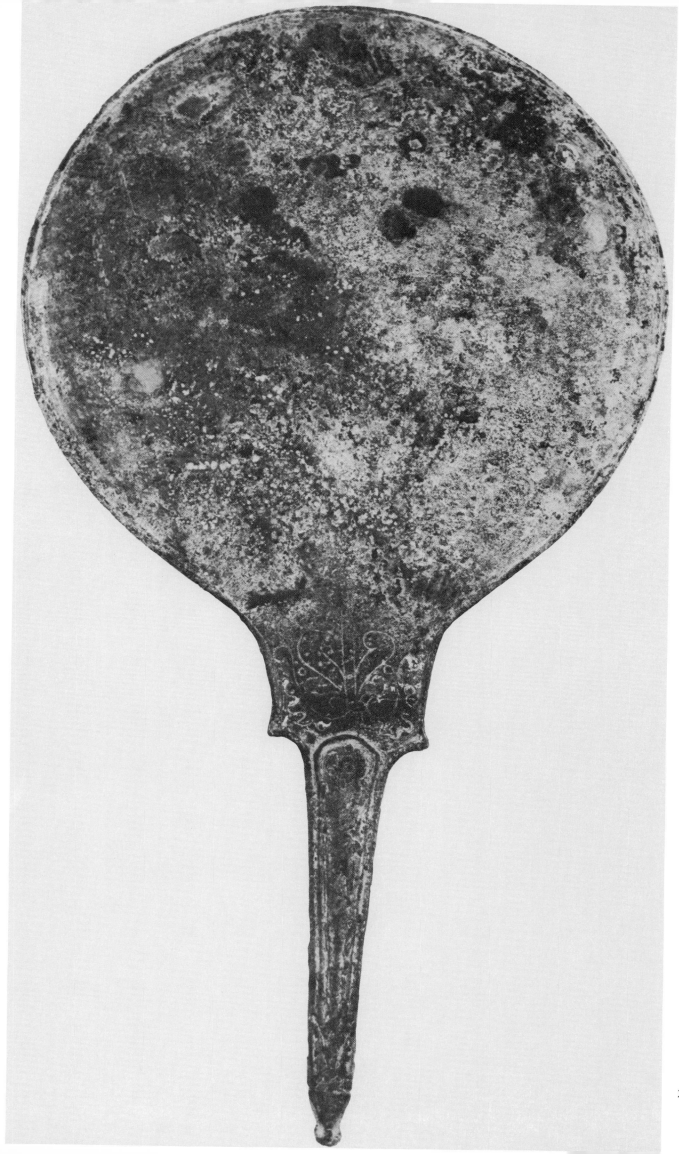

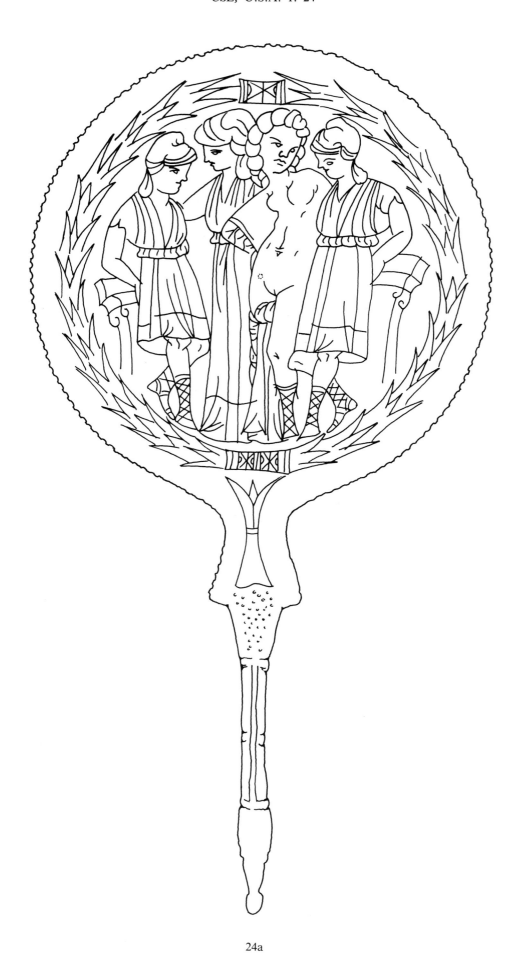

24a

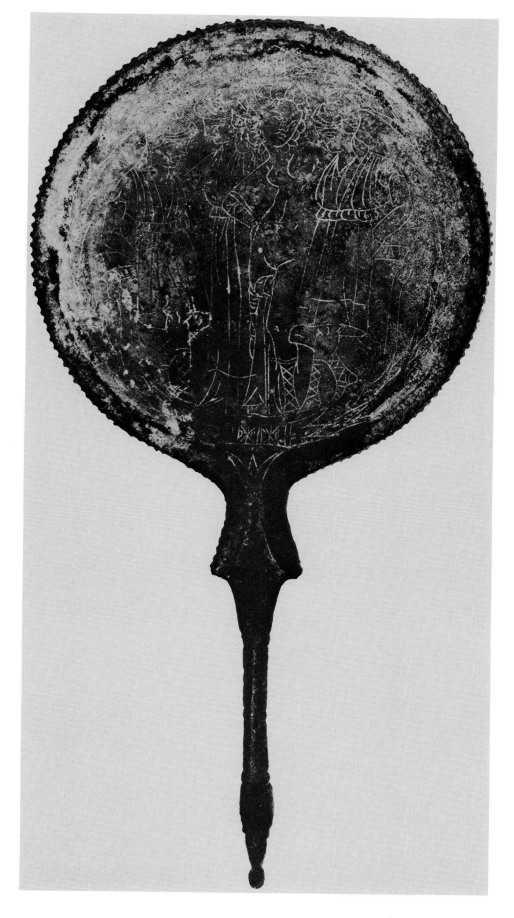

24b

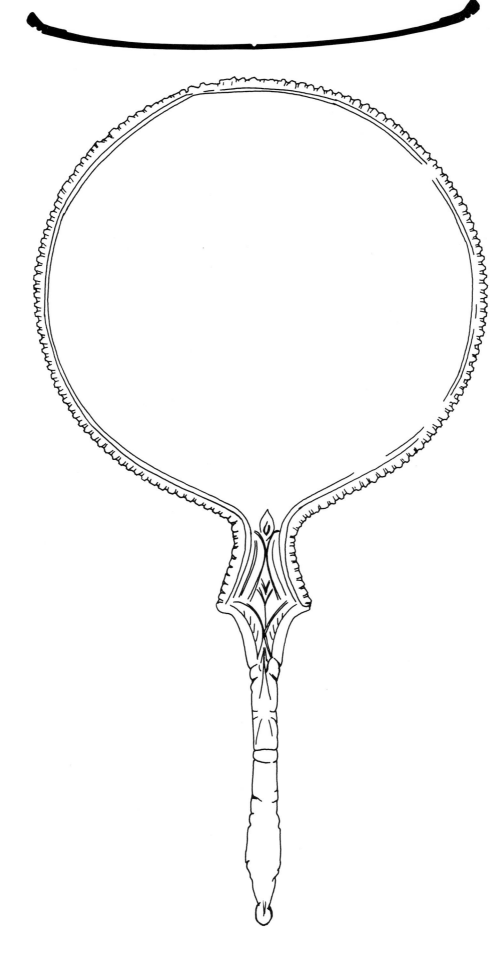

24c

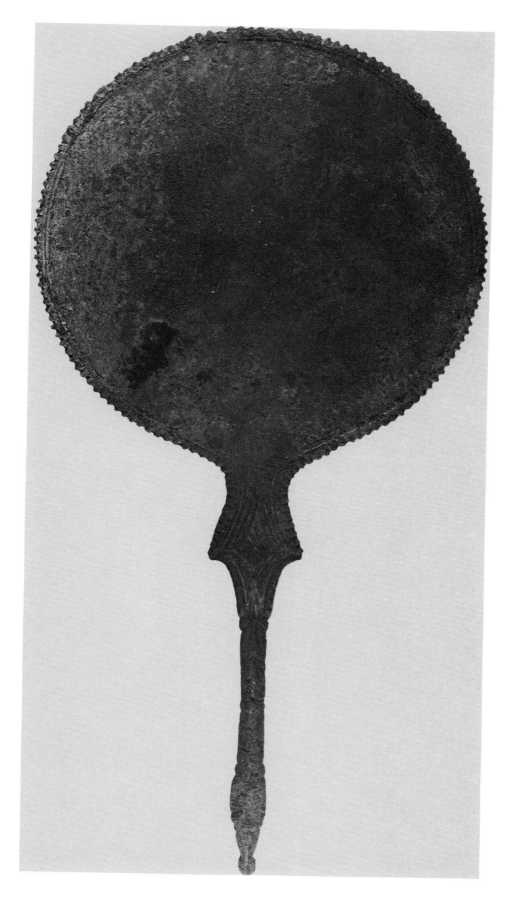

24d

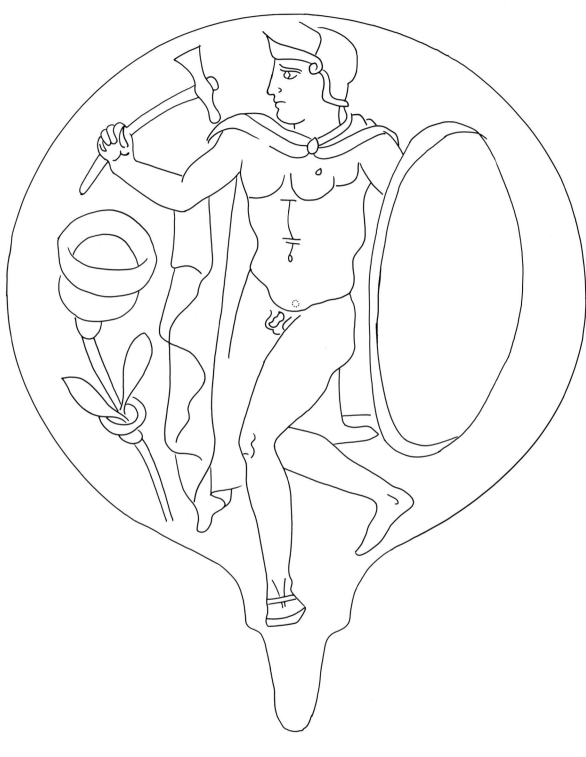

25a

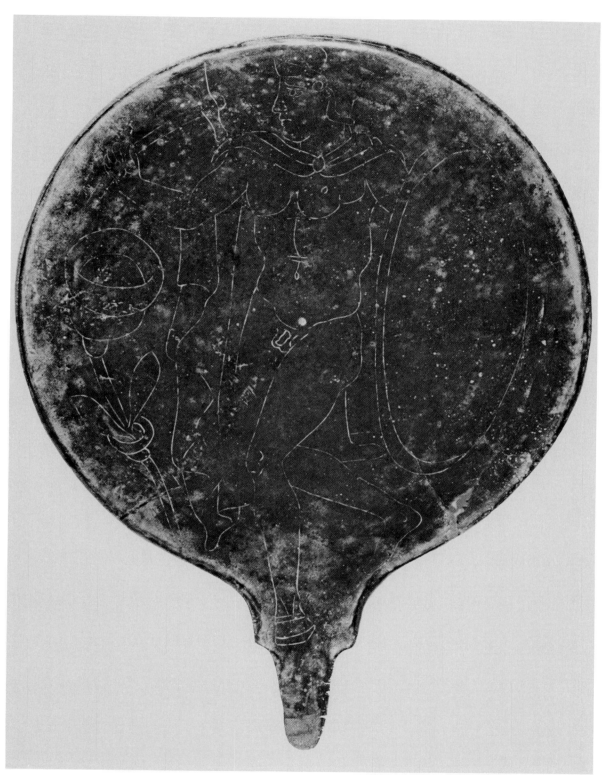

25b

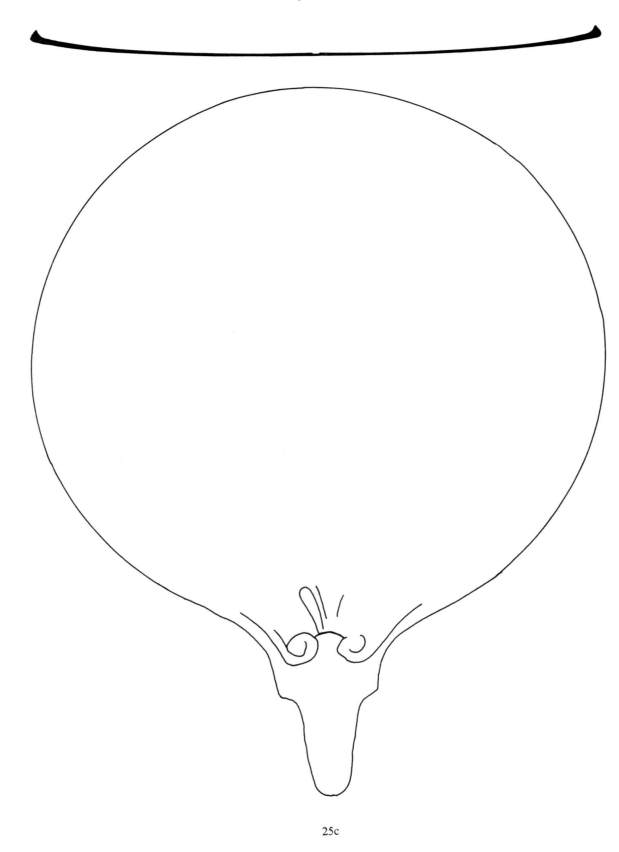

25c

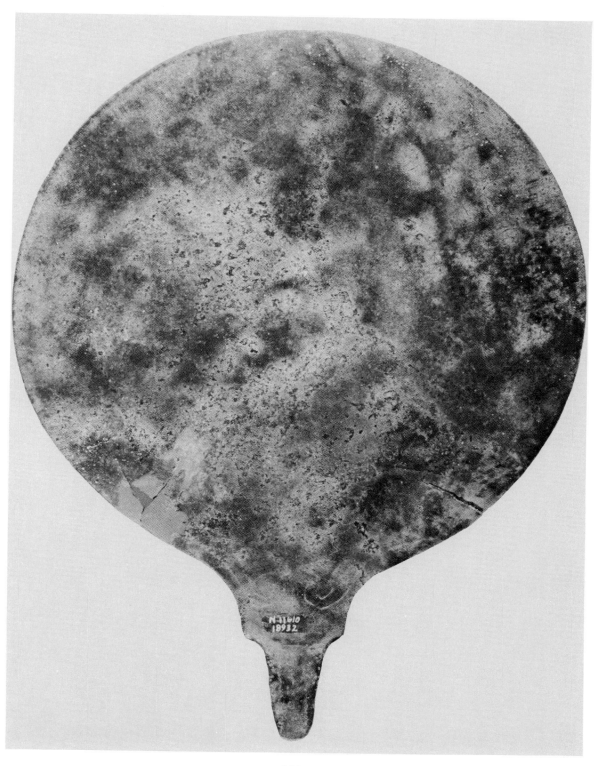

25d

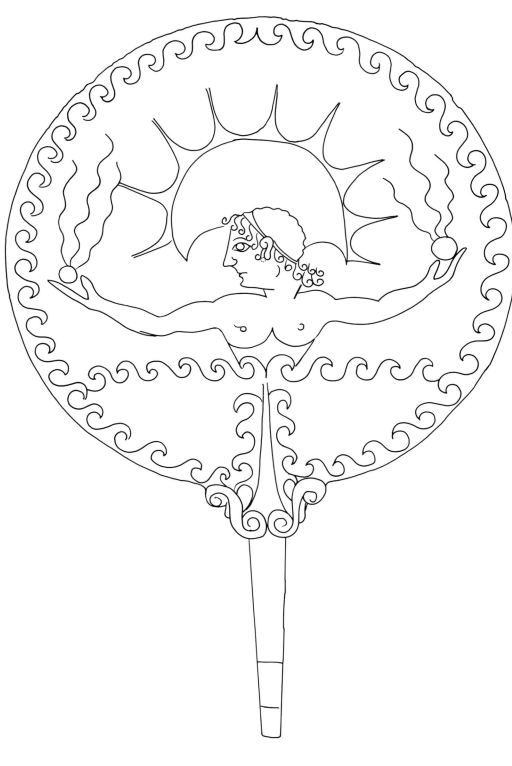

26a

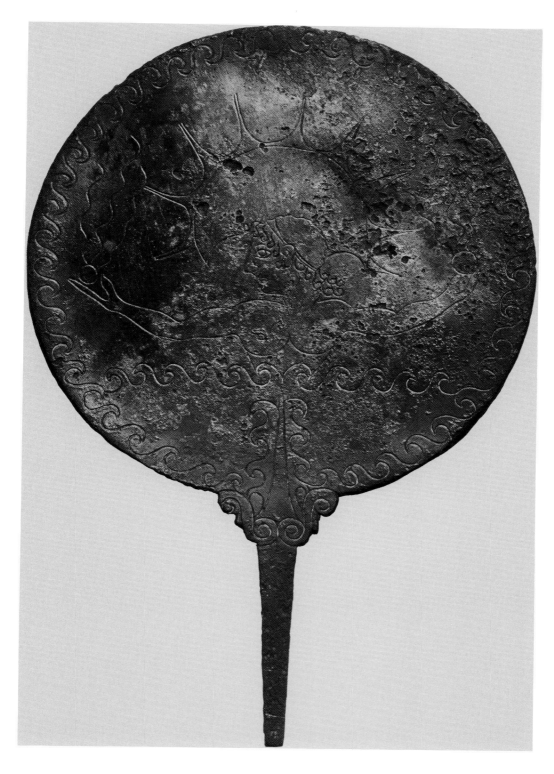

26b

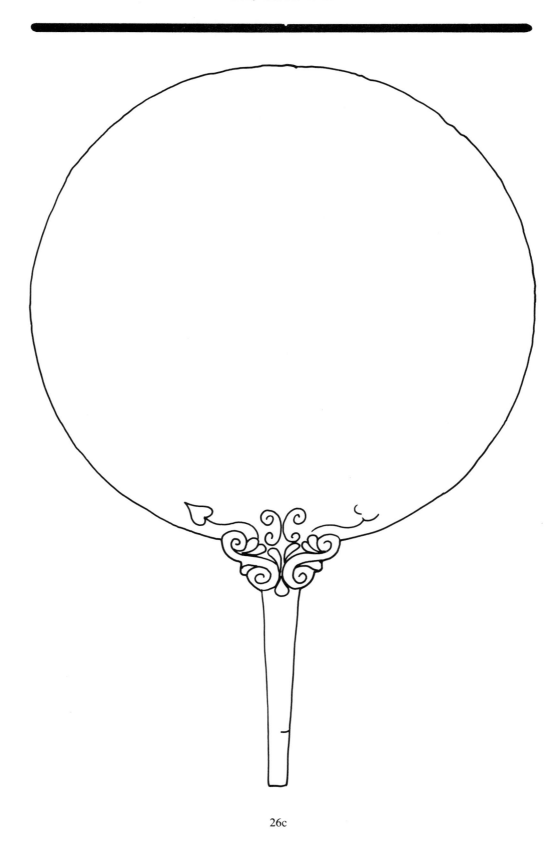

26c

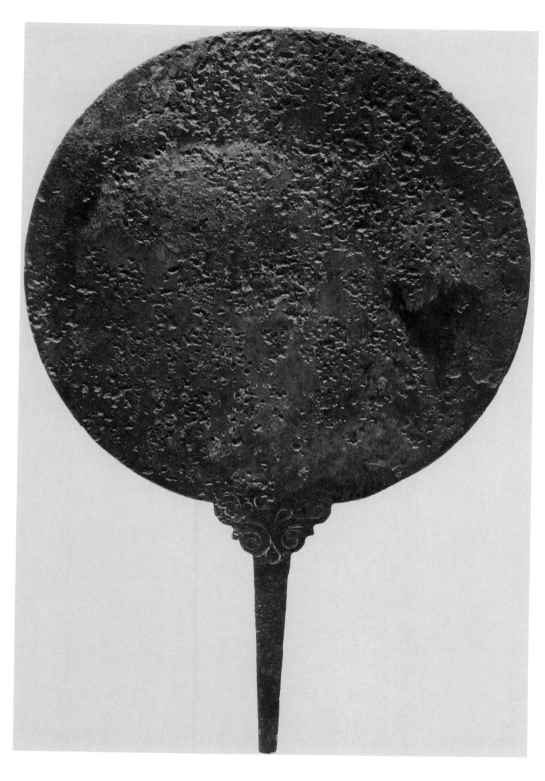

26d

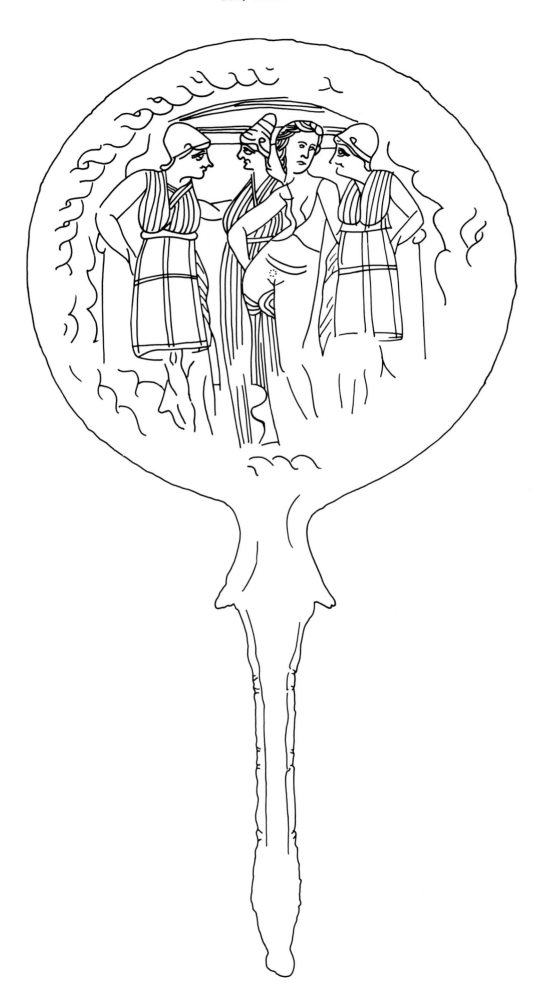

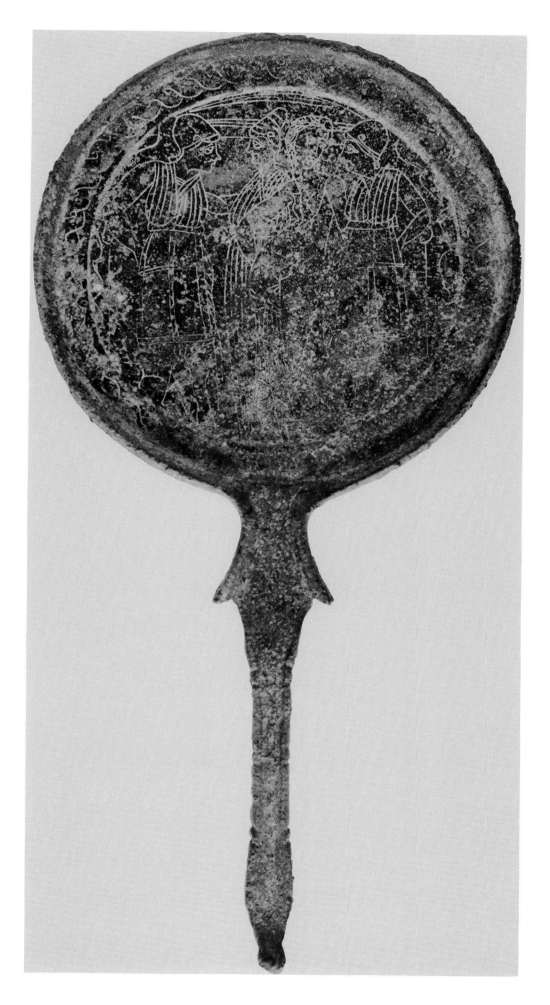

27b

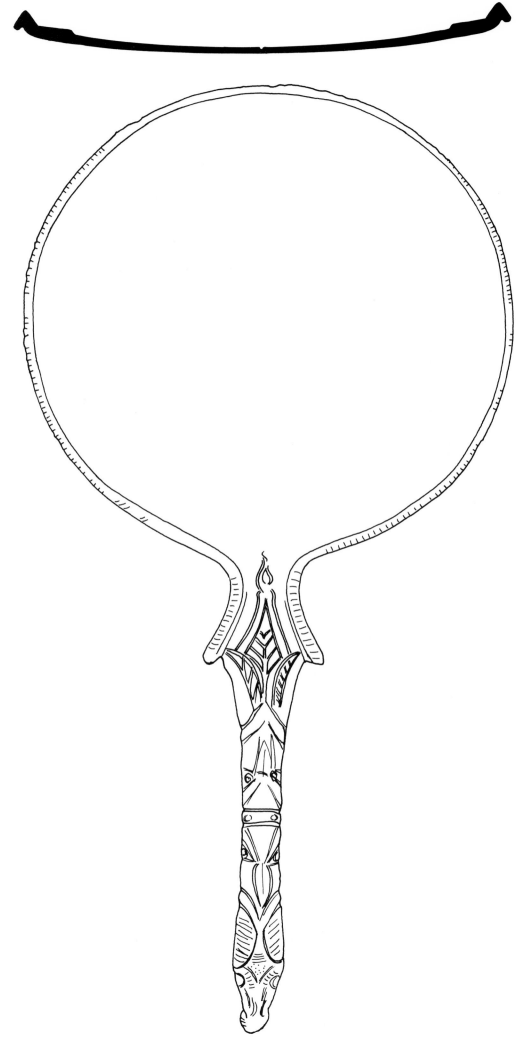

27c

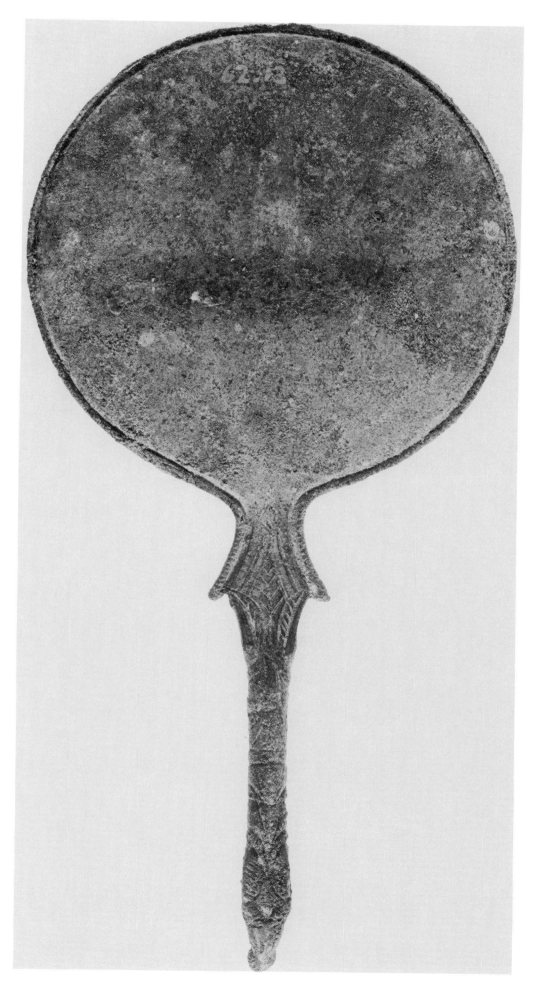

27d

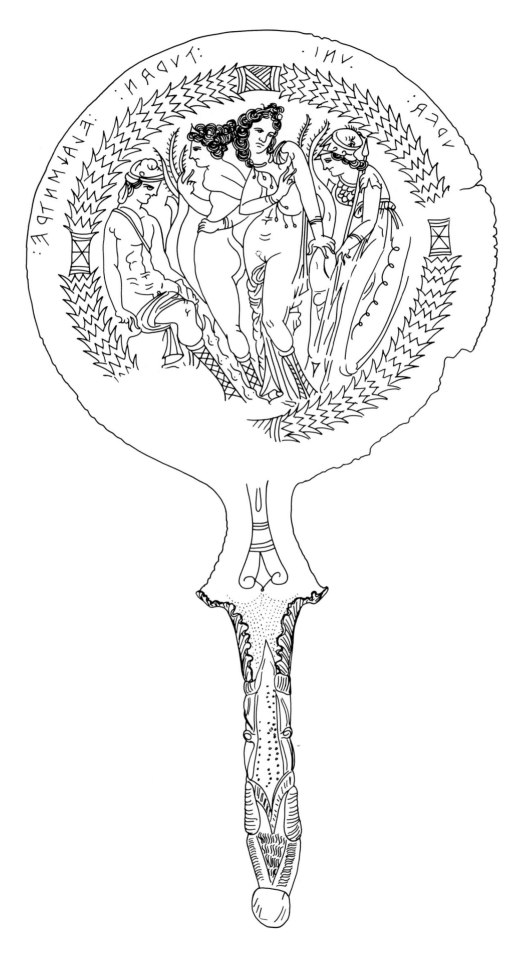

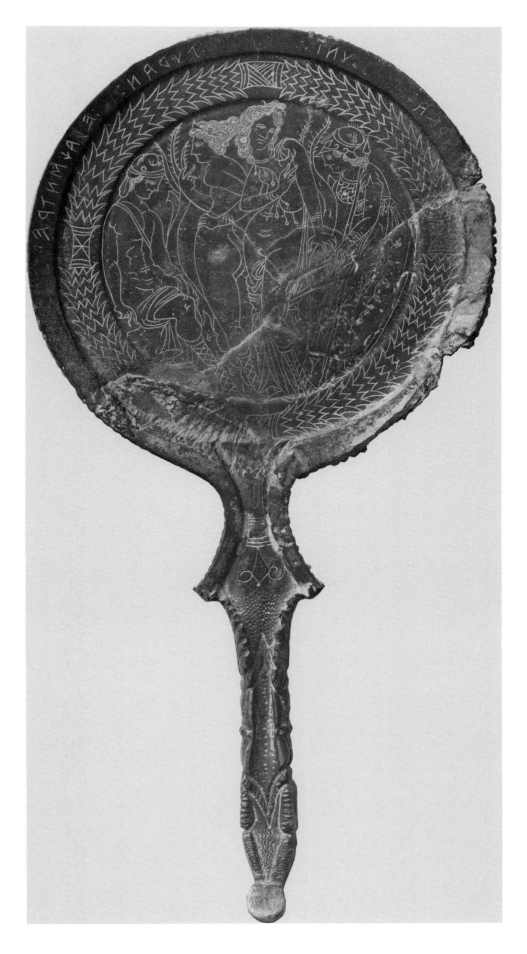

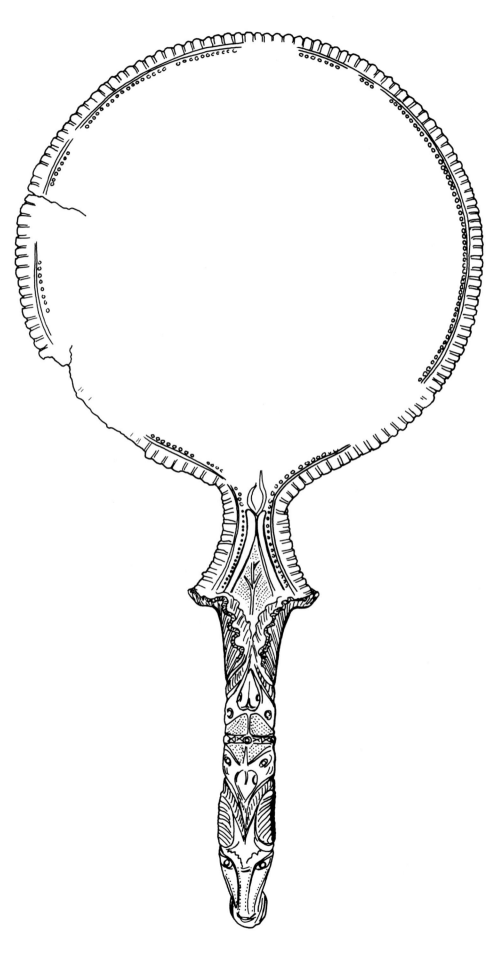

28c

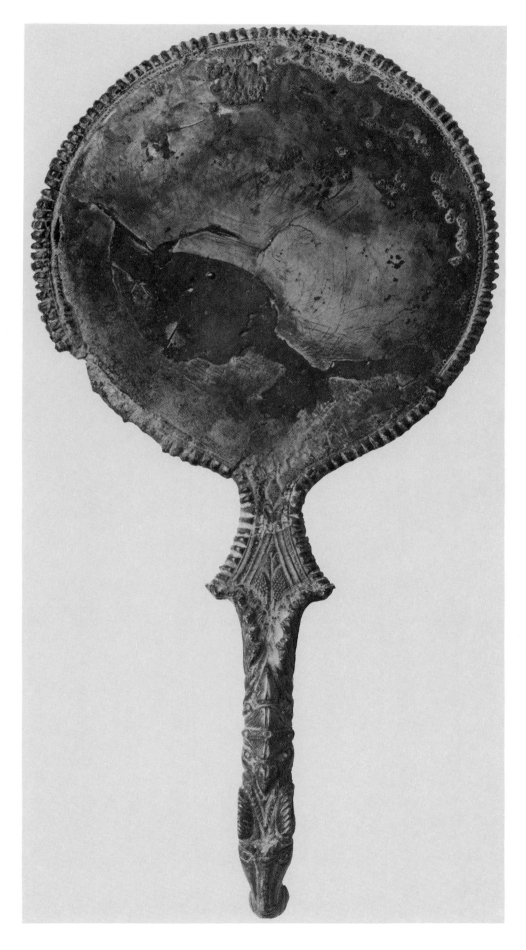

28d

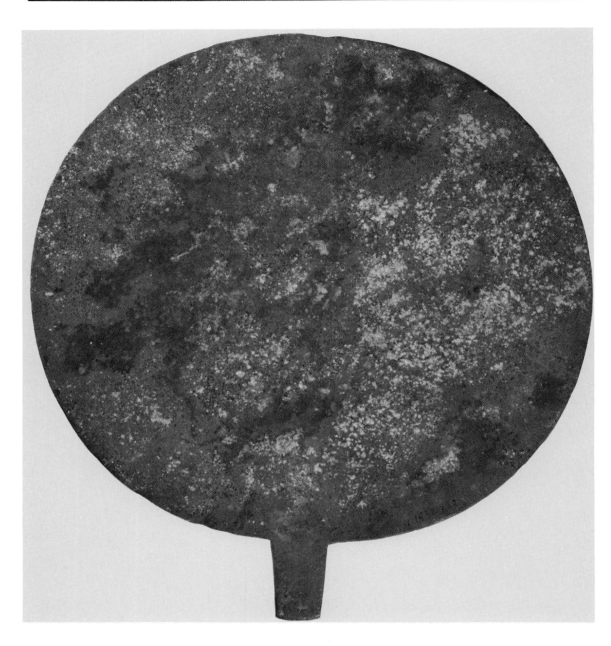

29a

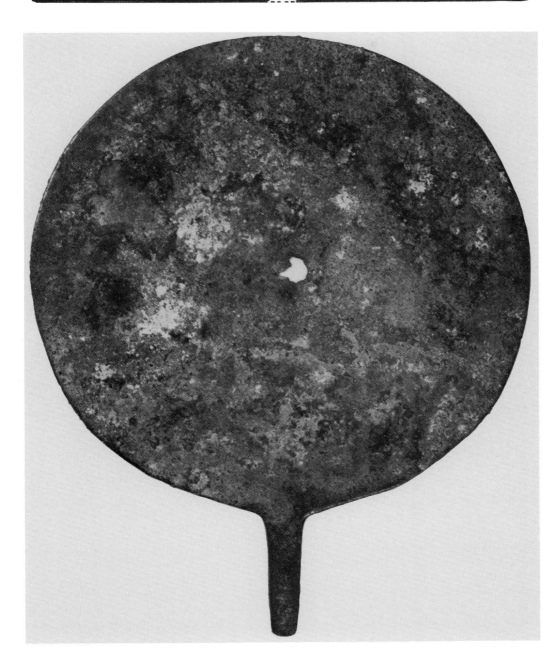

30a

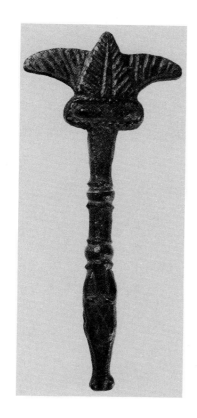

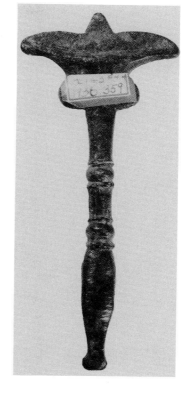

31a   31b

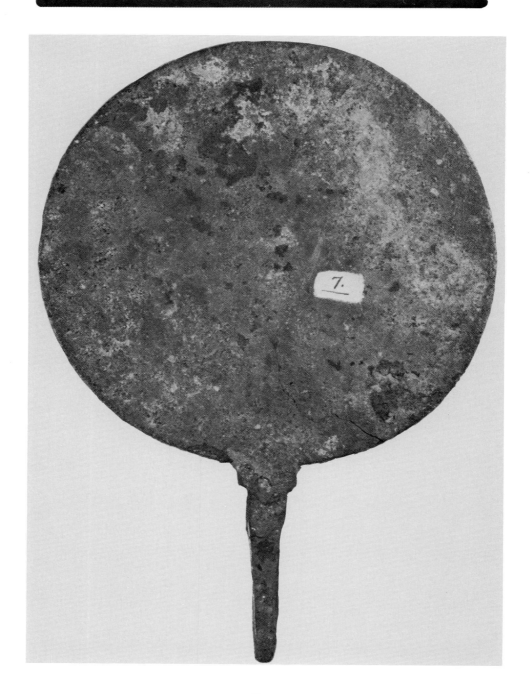

32a

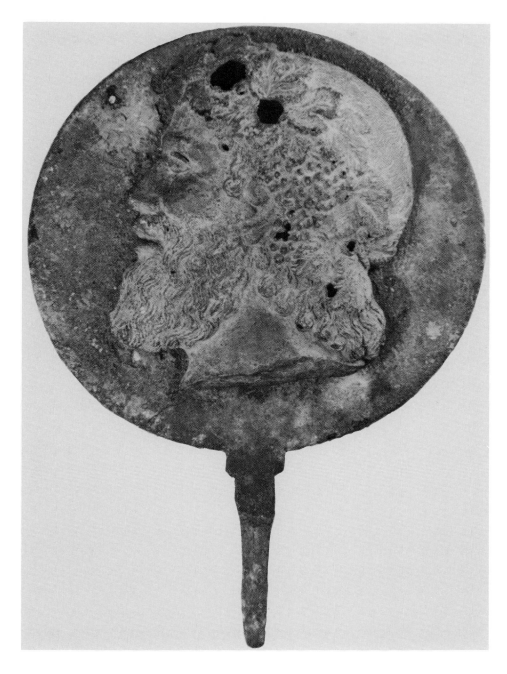

32b

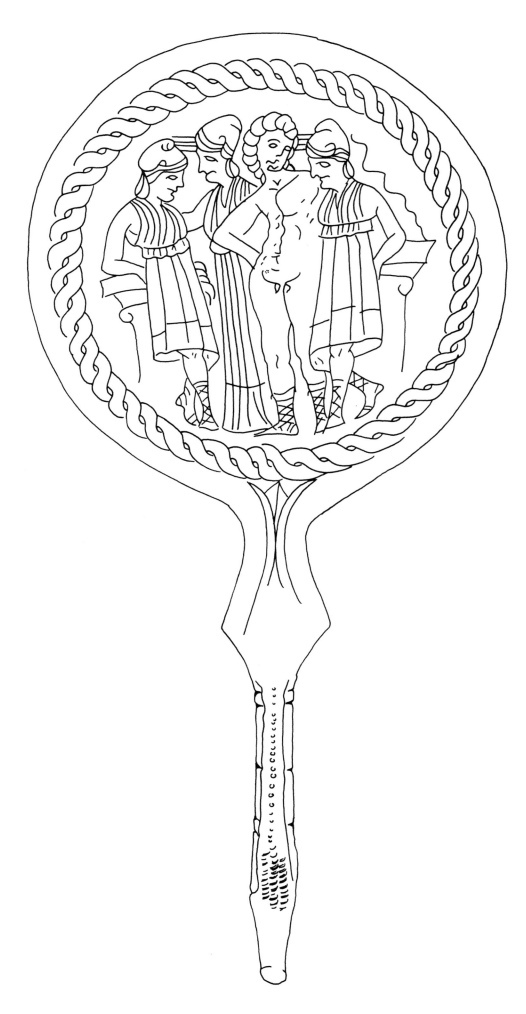

33a

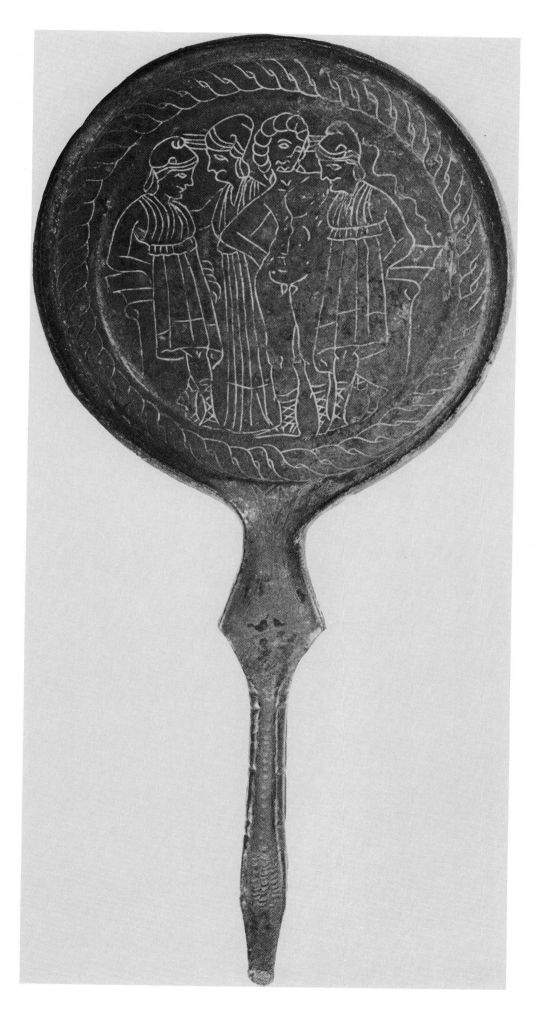

33b

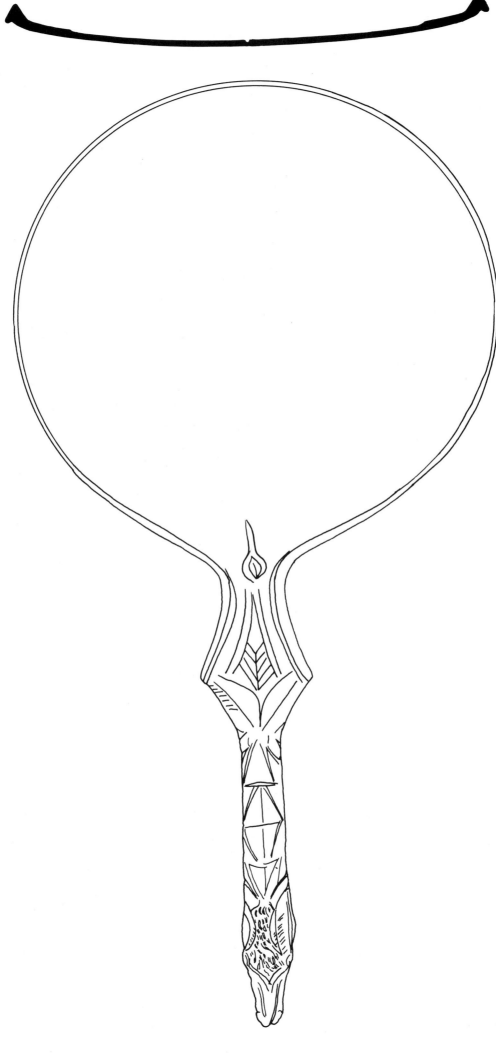

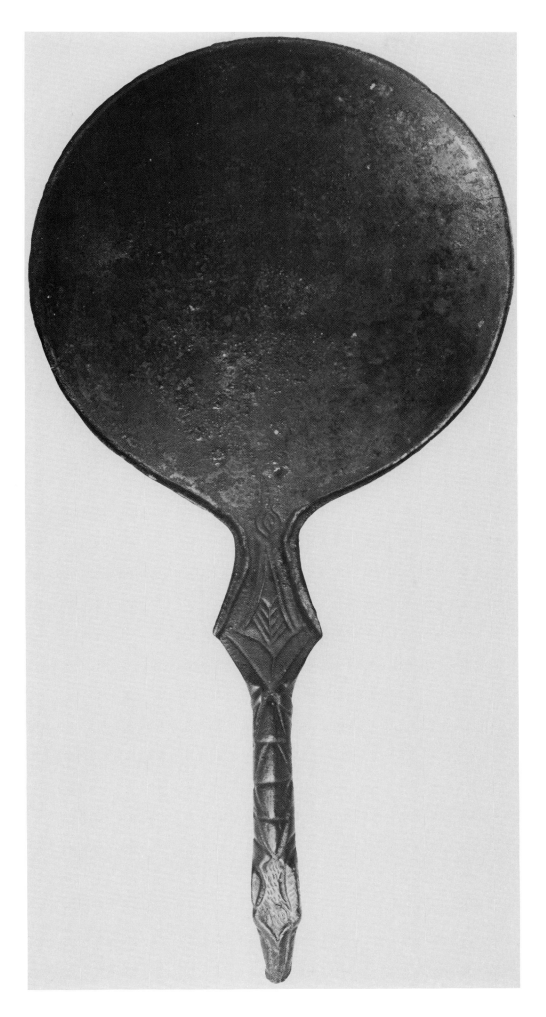

33d

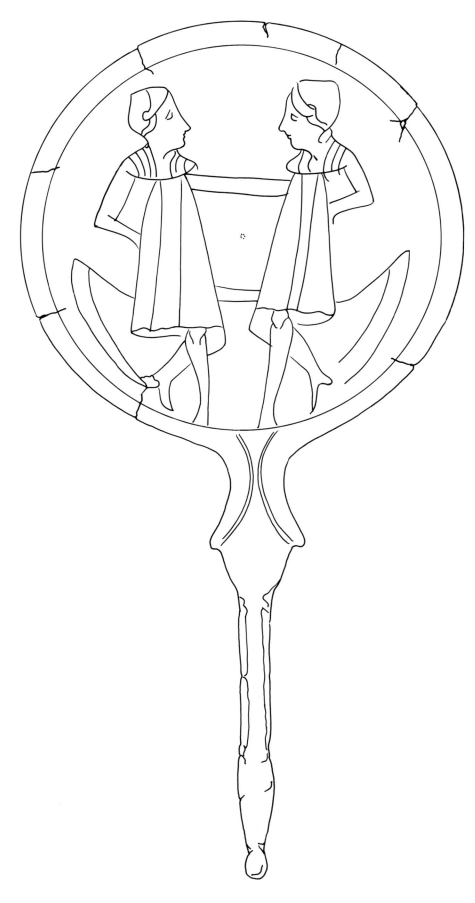

34a

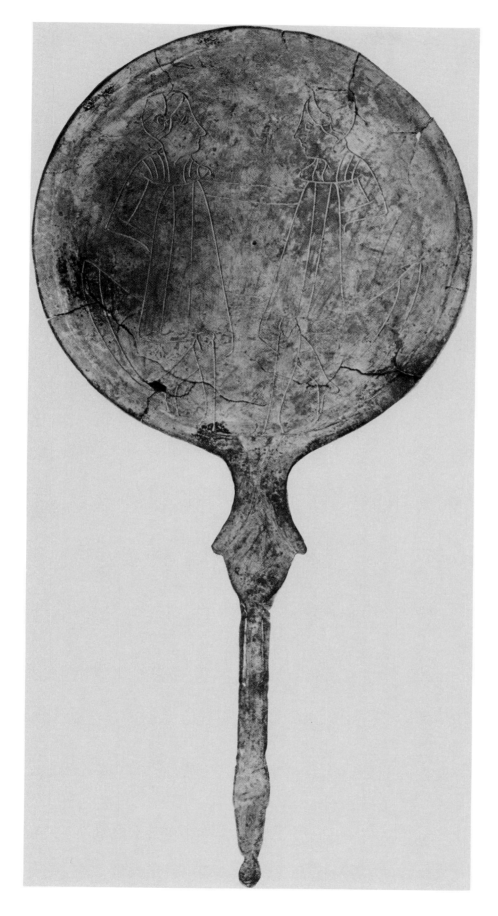

34b.

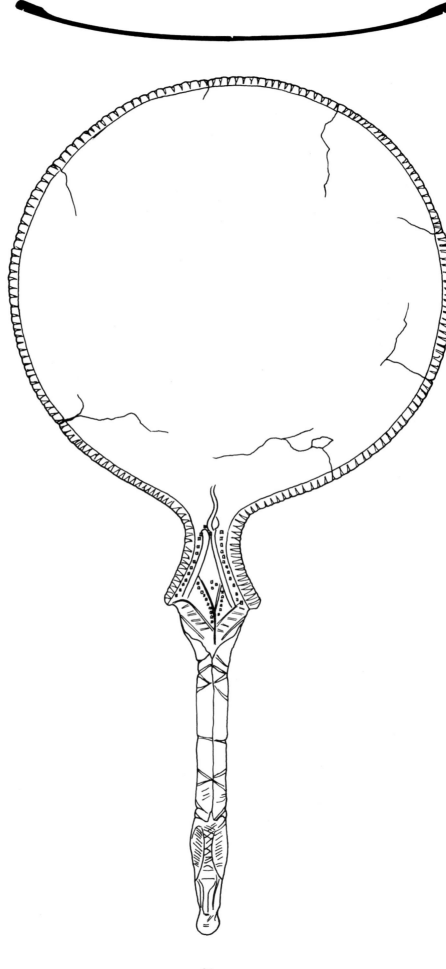

34c

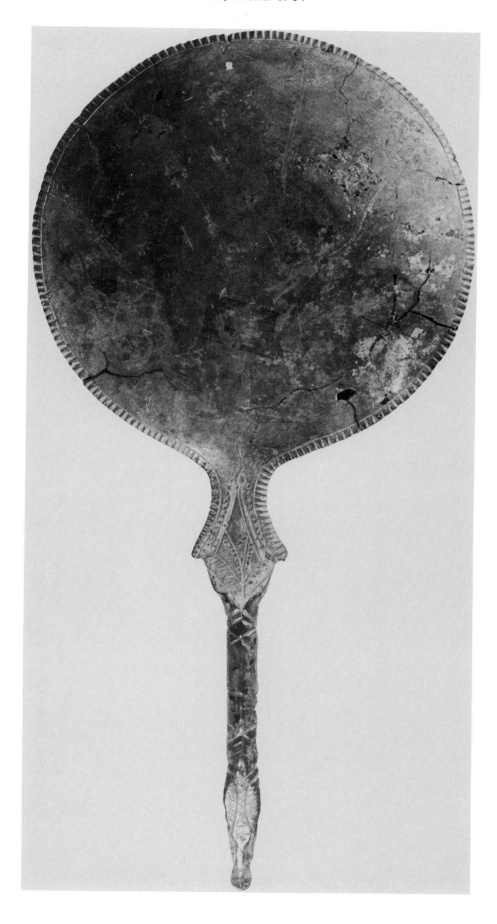

34d

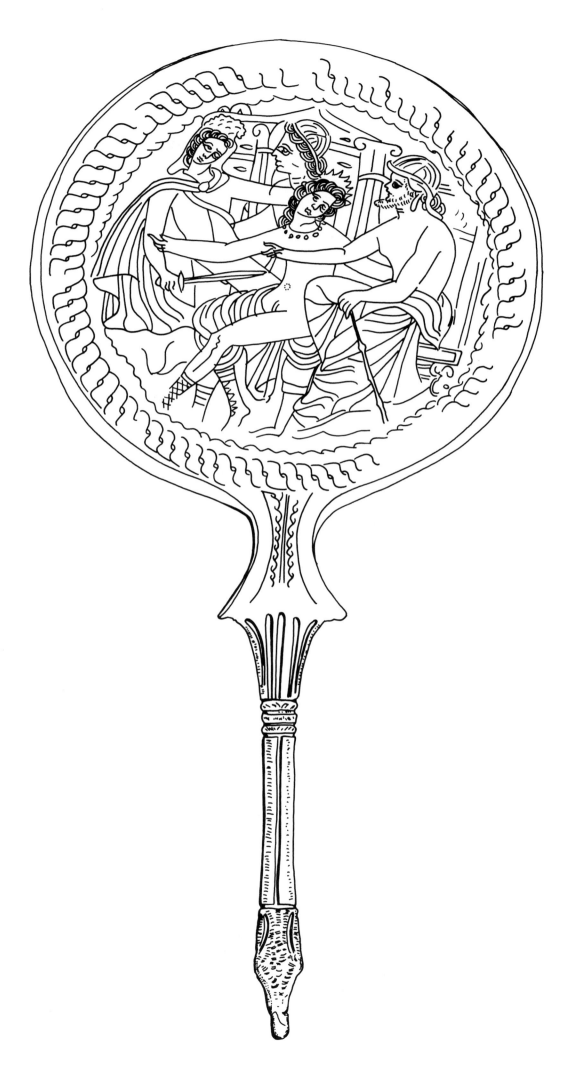

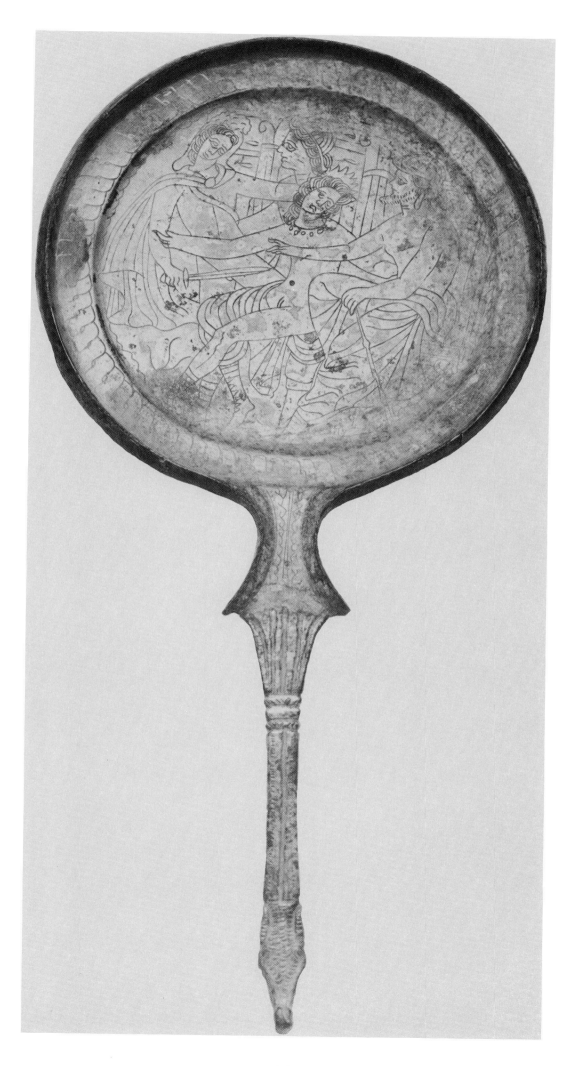

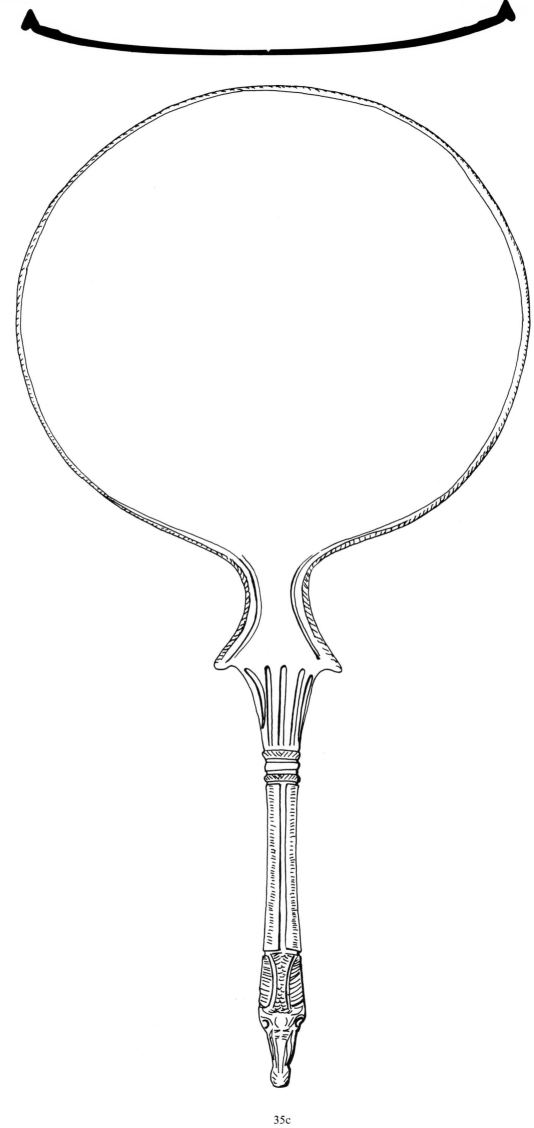

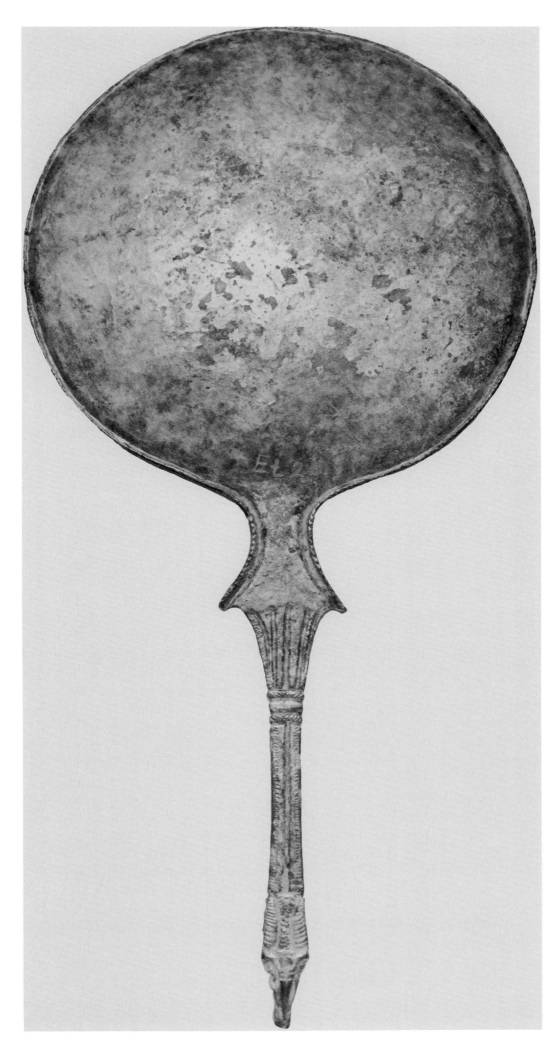

35d

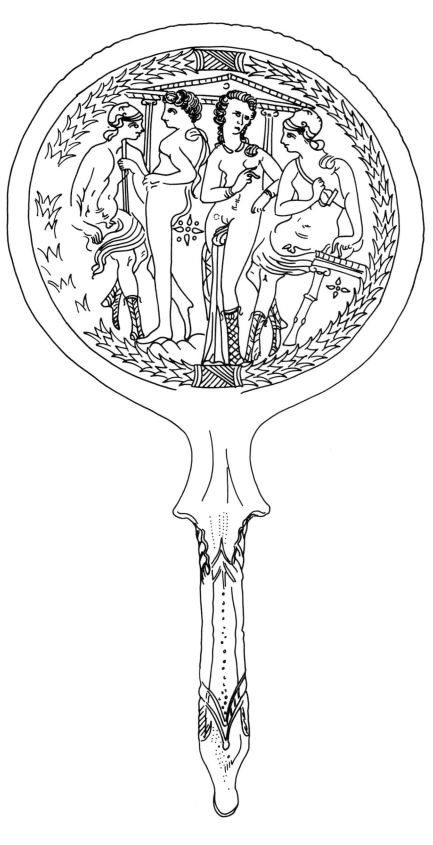

36a

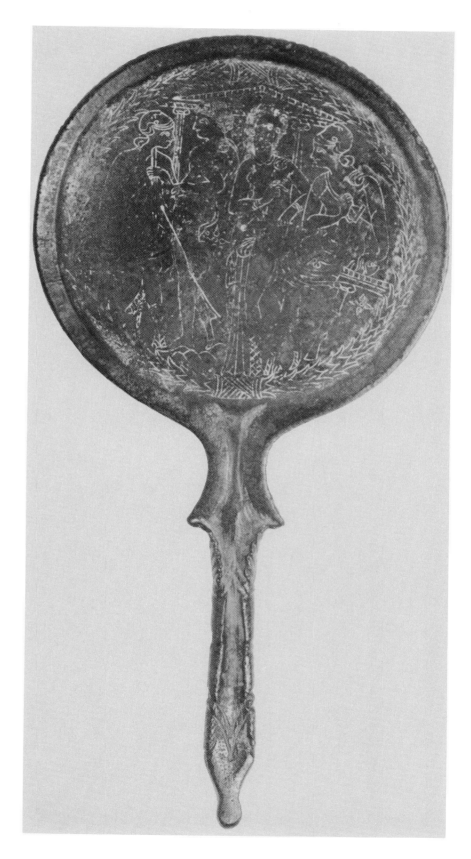

36b

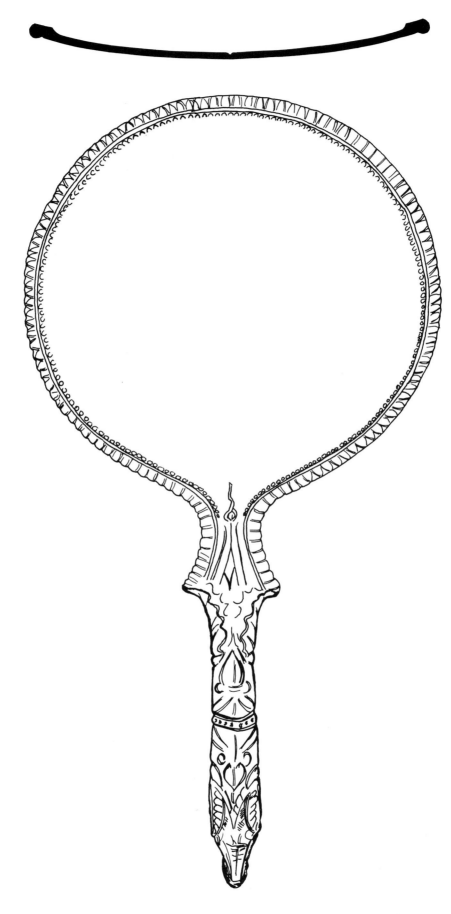

36c

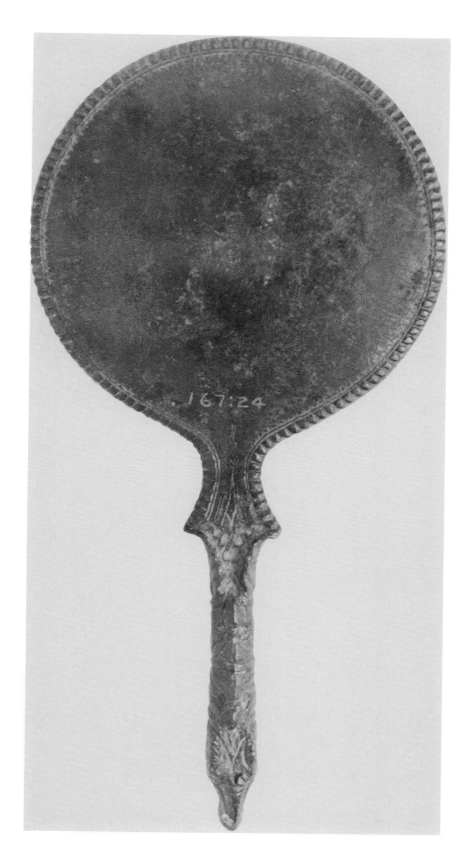

36d

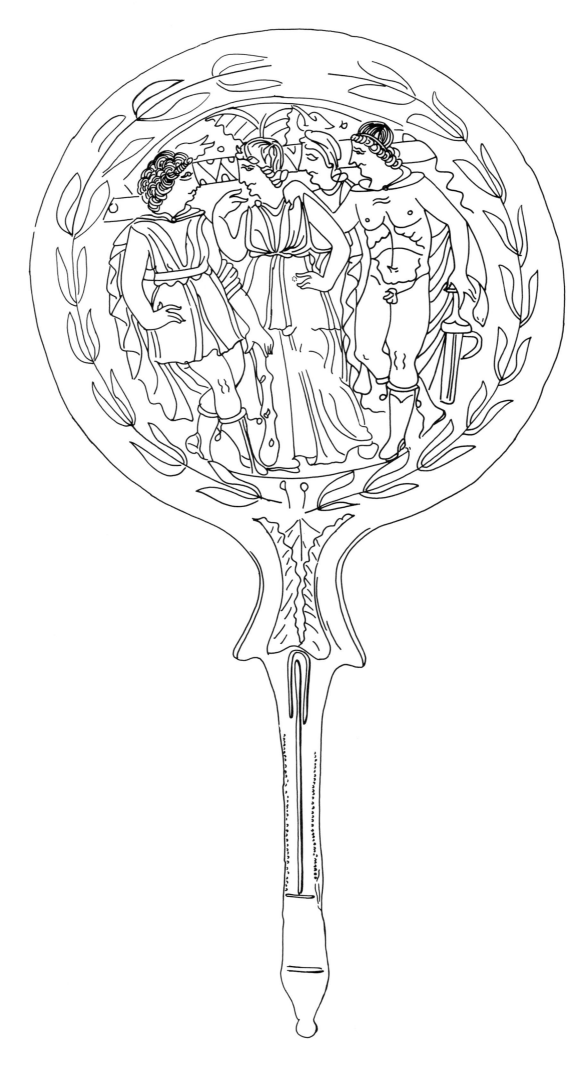

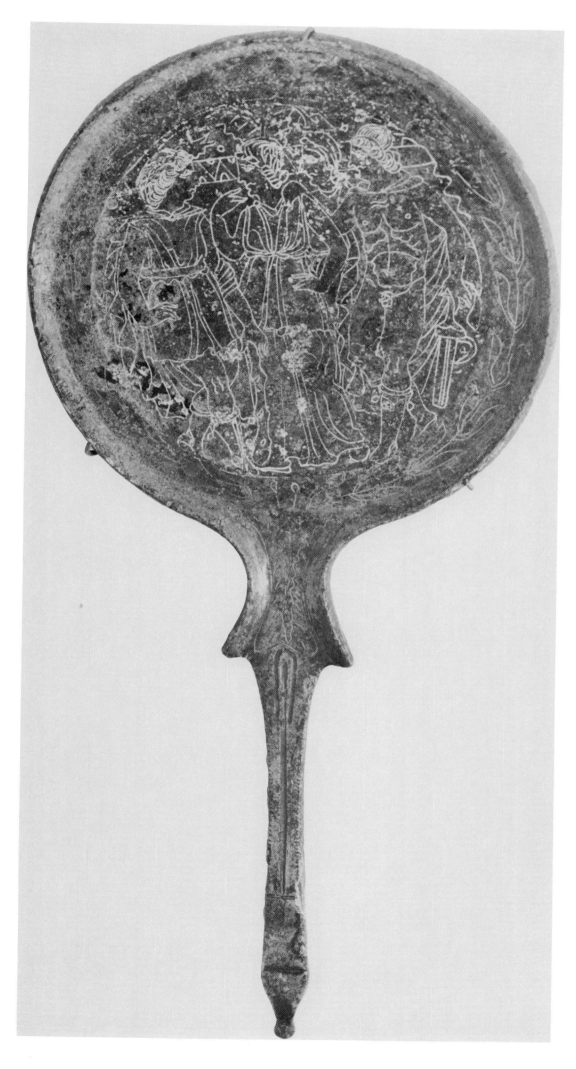

204

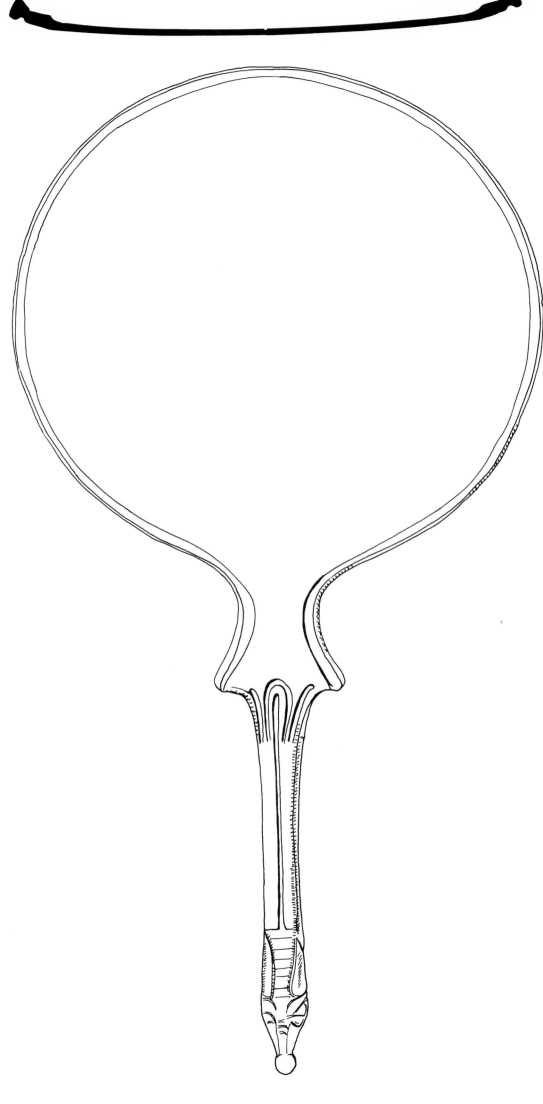

37c

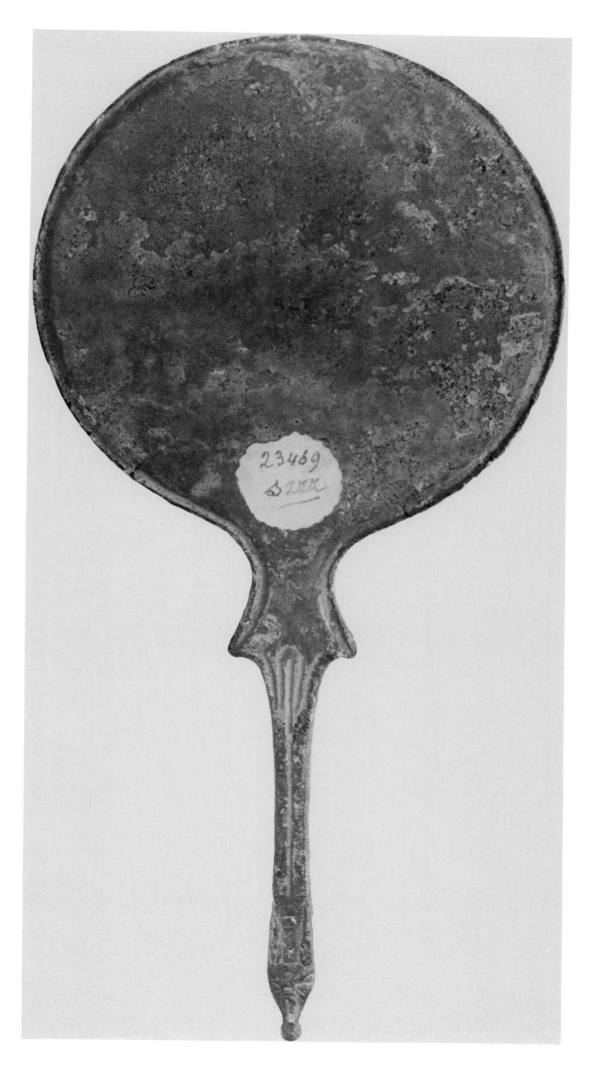

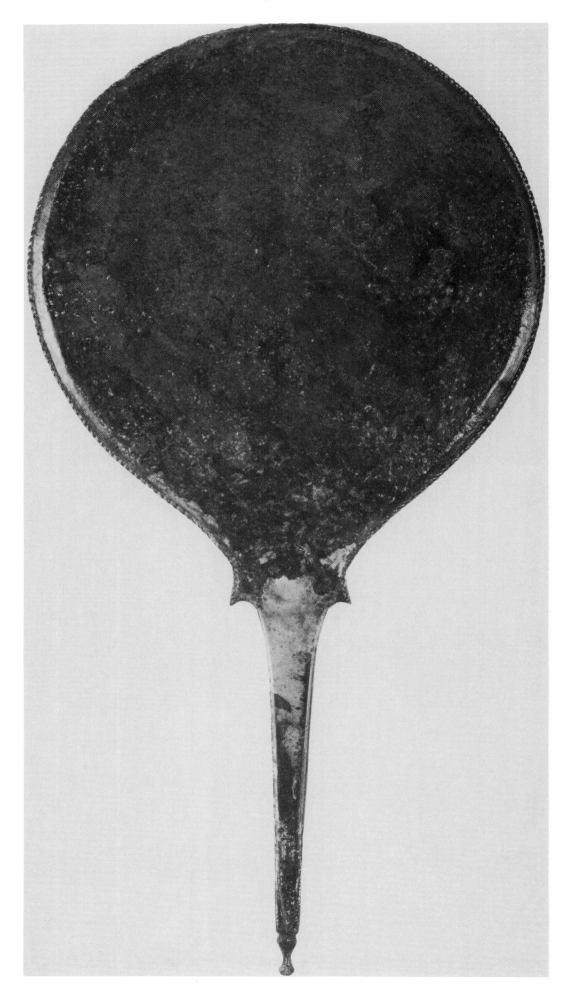

38a

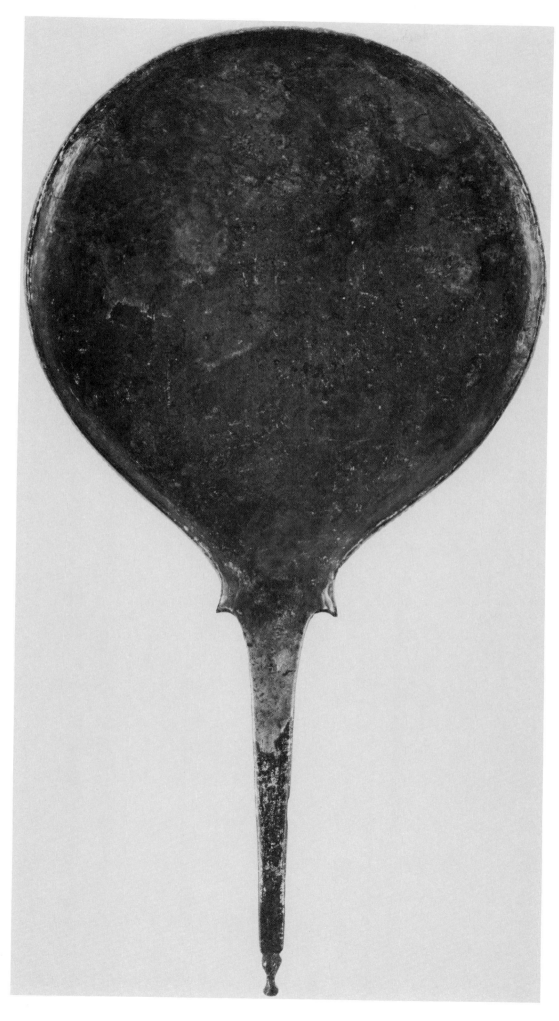

38b

208

ΠΟΛΟΥCEΣ

CASTOR

AMVCOS

39a

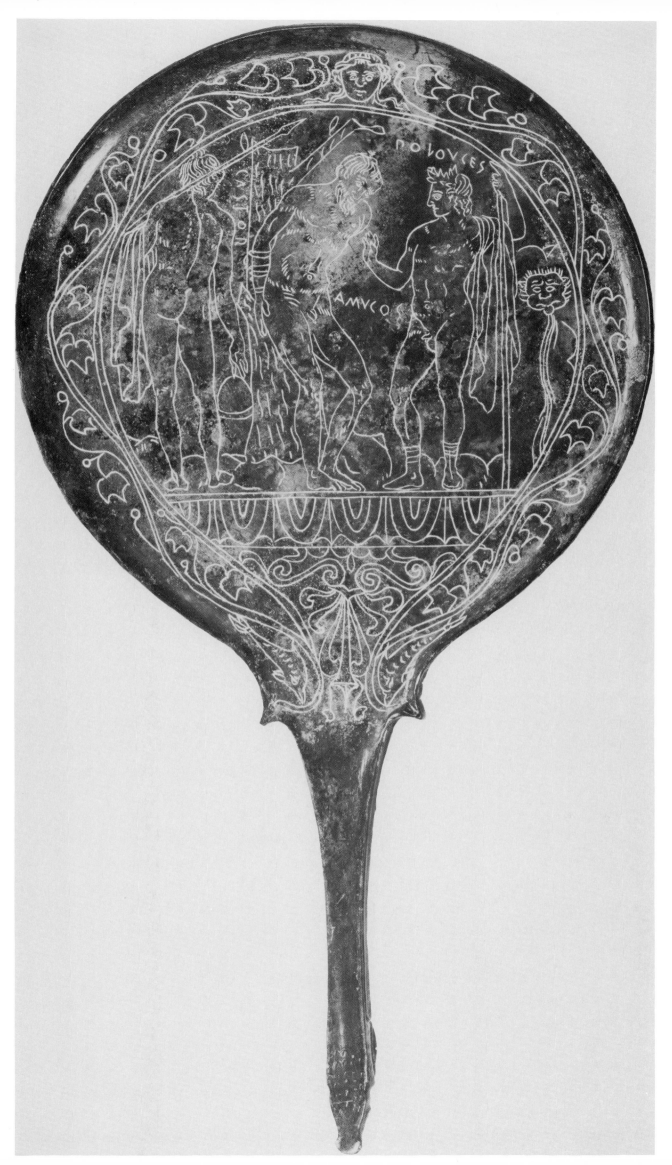

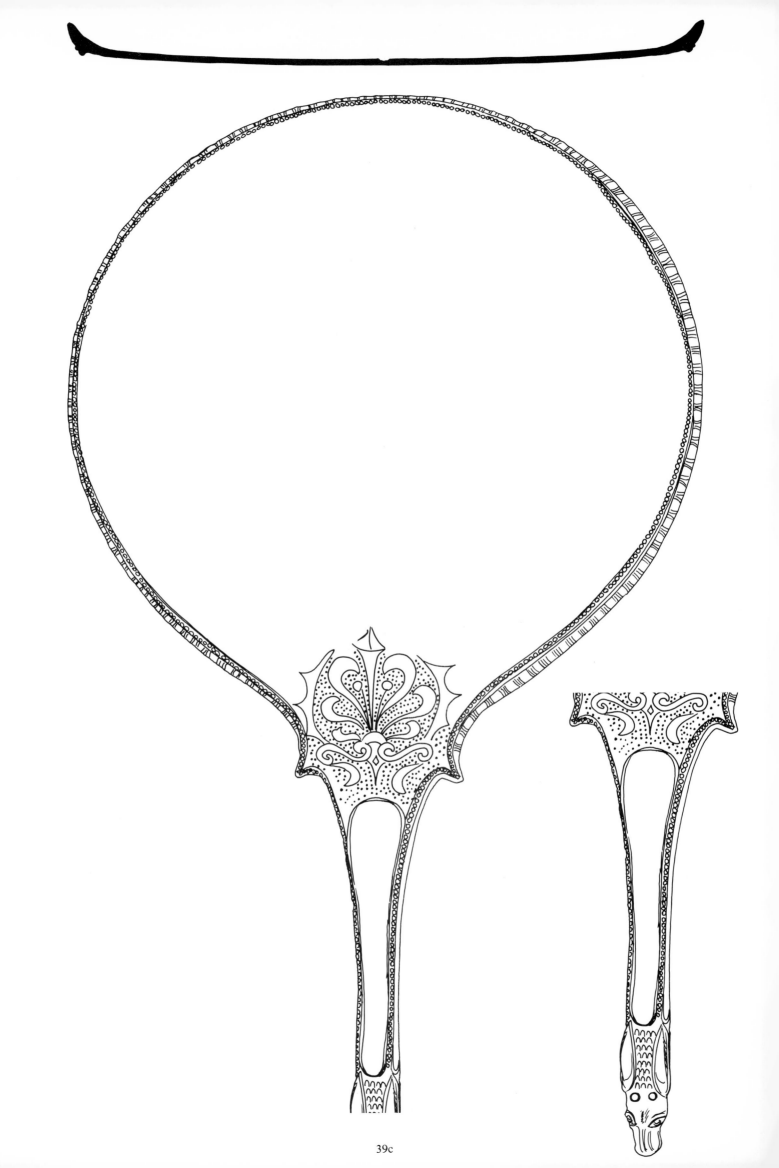

39c

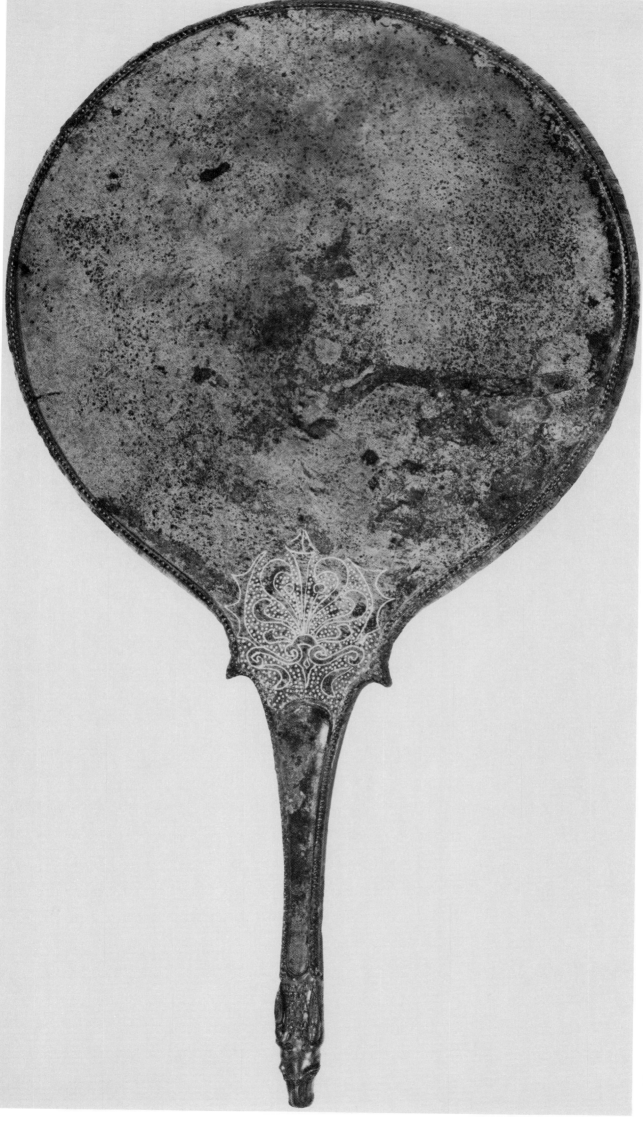

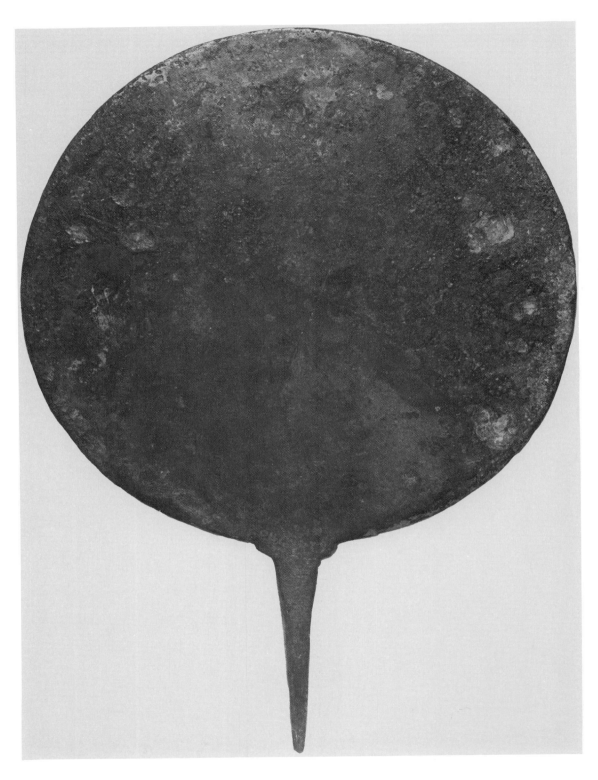

40a

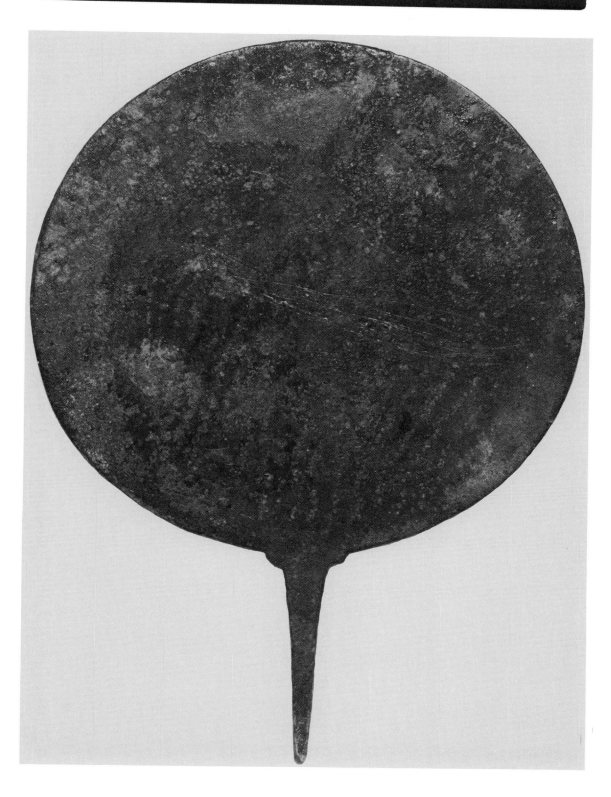

40b

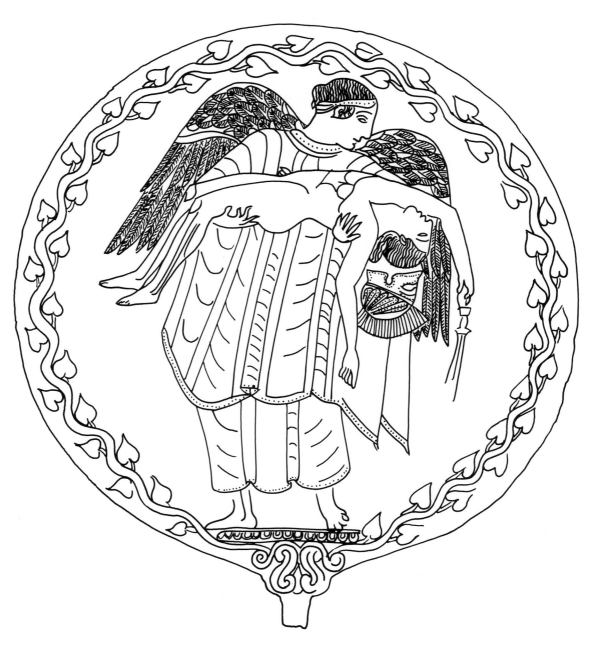

41a

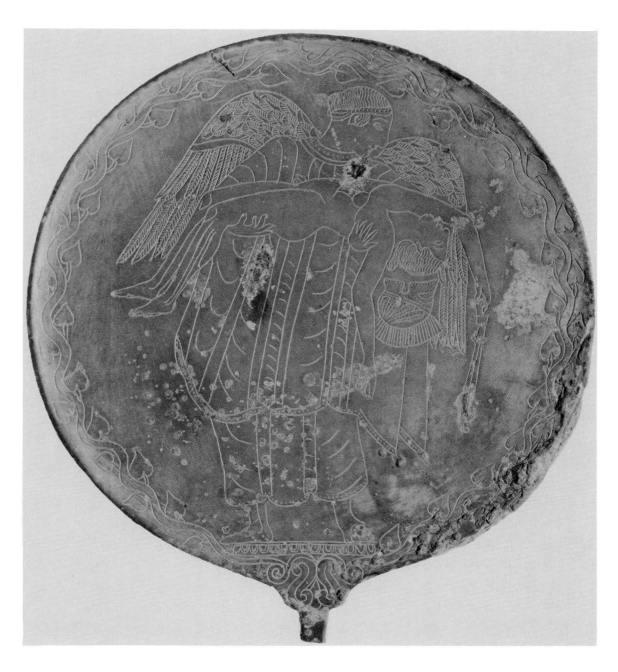

41b

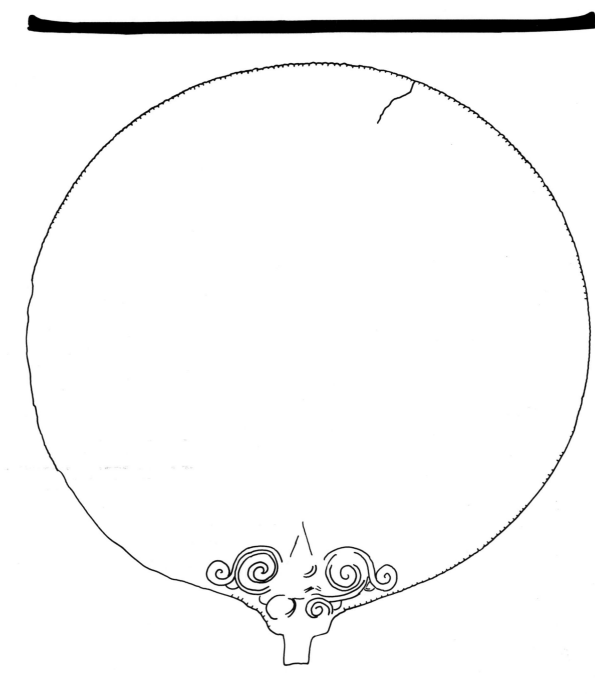

41c

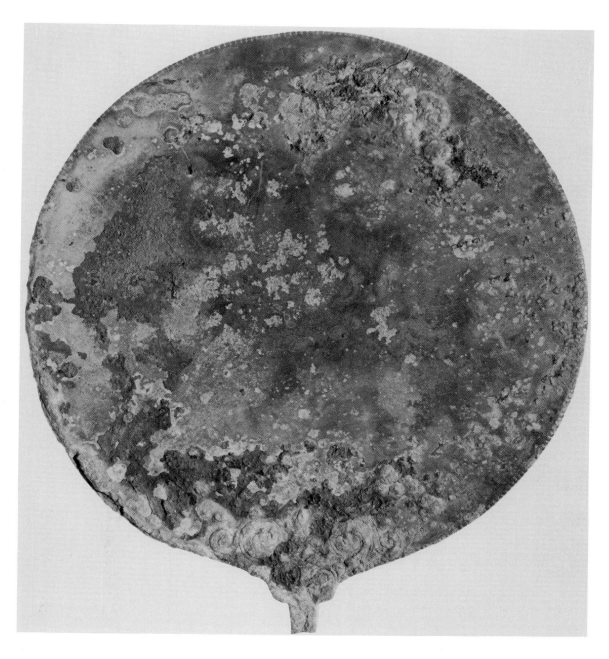

41d

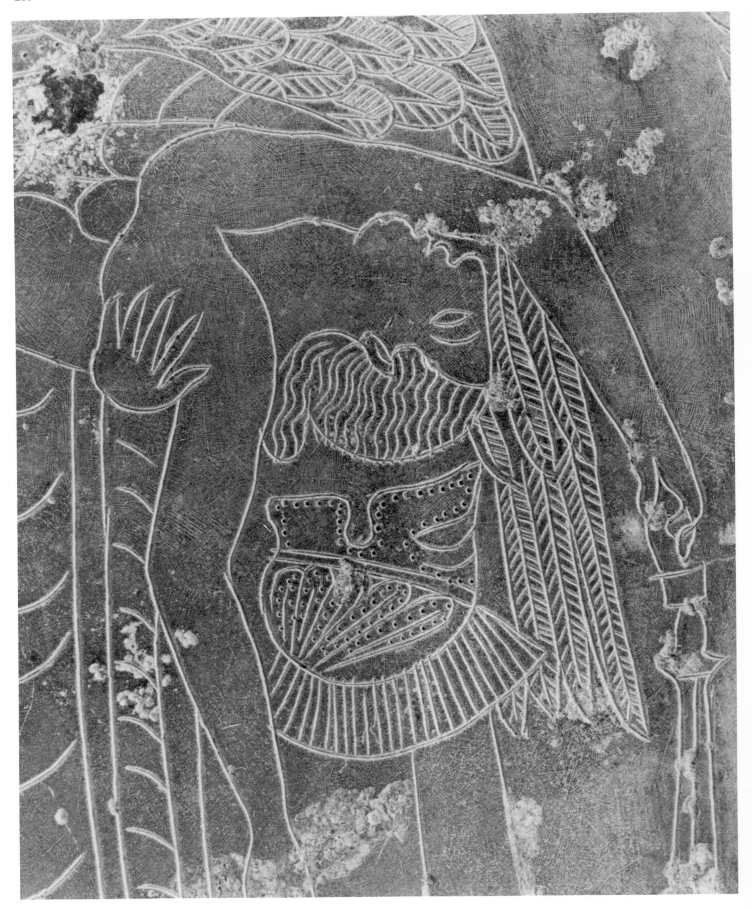

41e

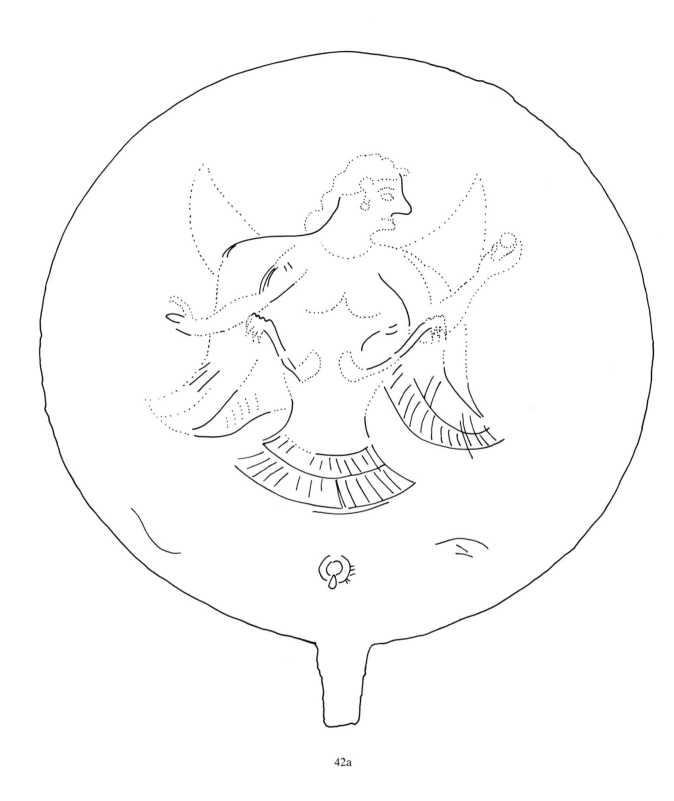

42a

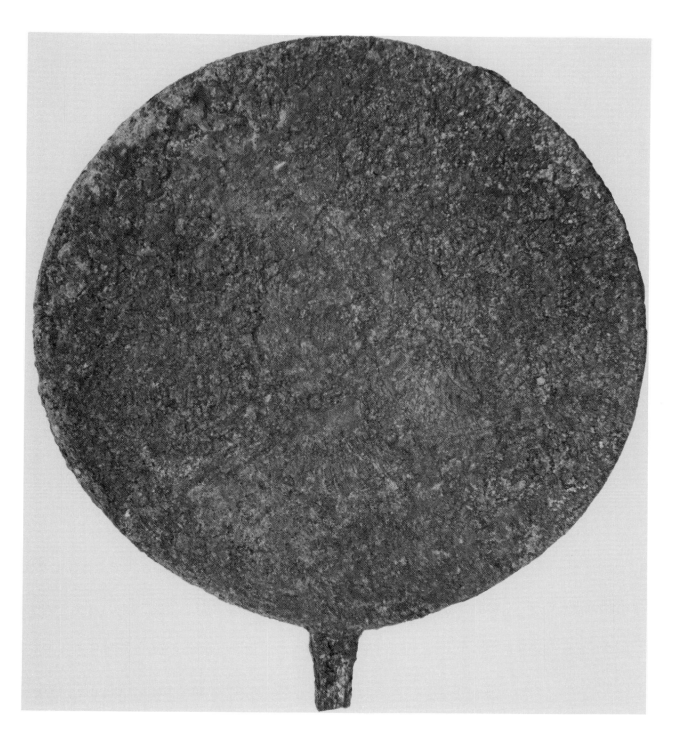

42b

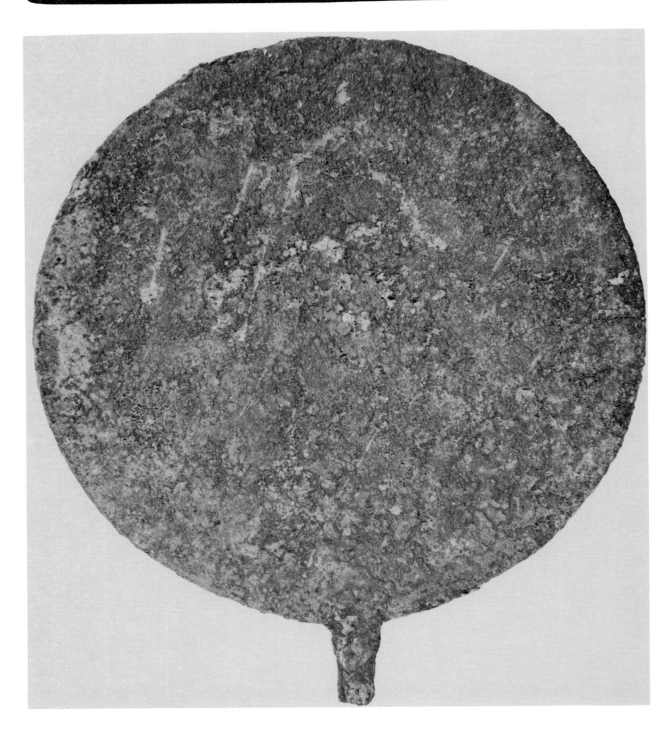

42c

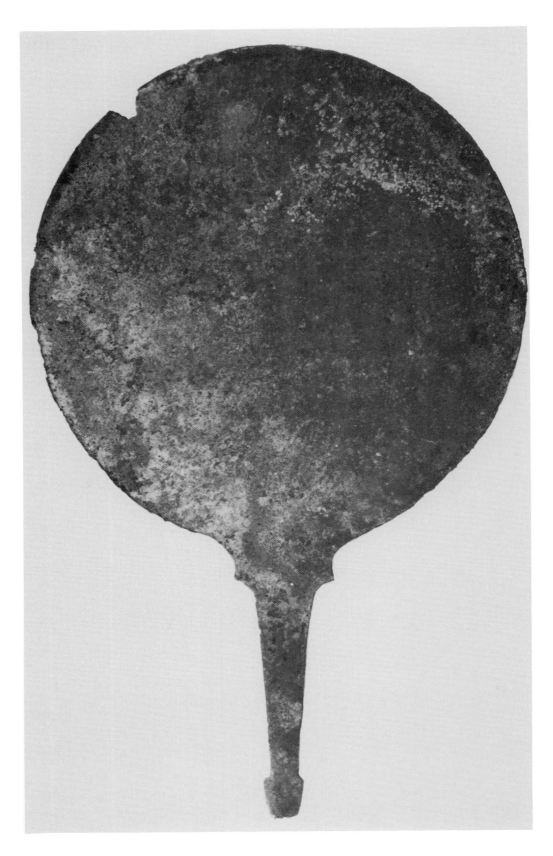

43a

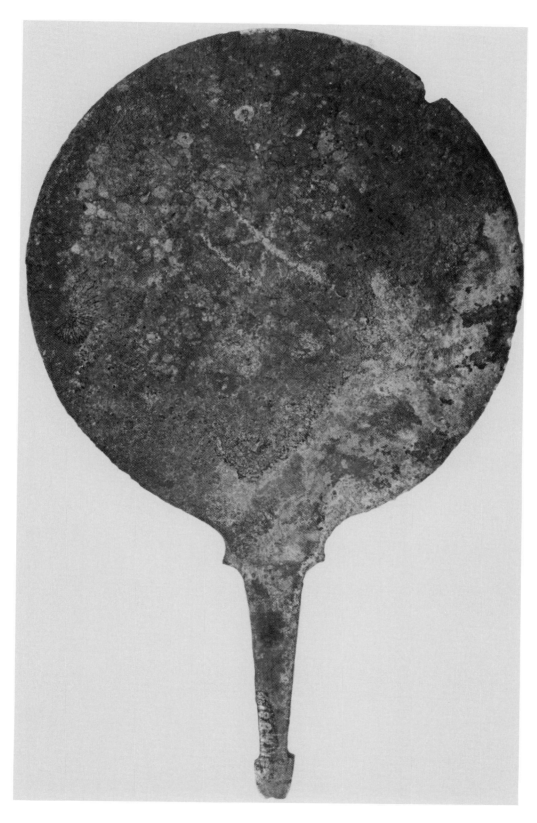

43b

44a

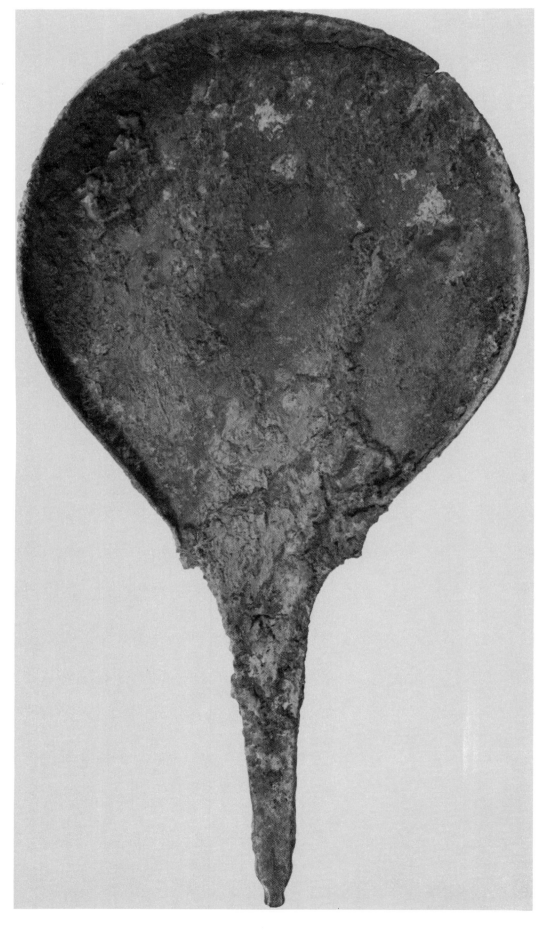

44a

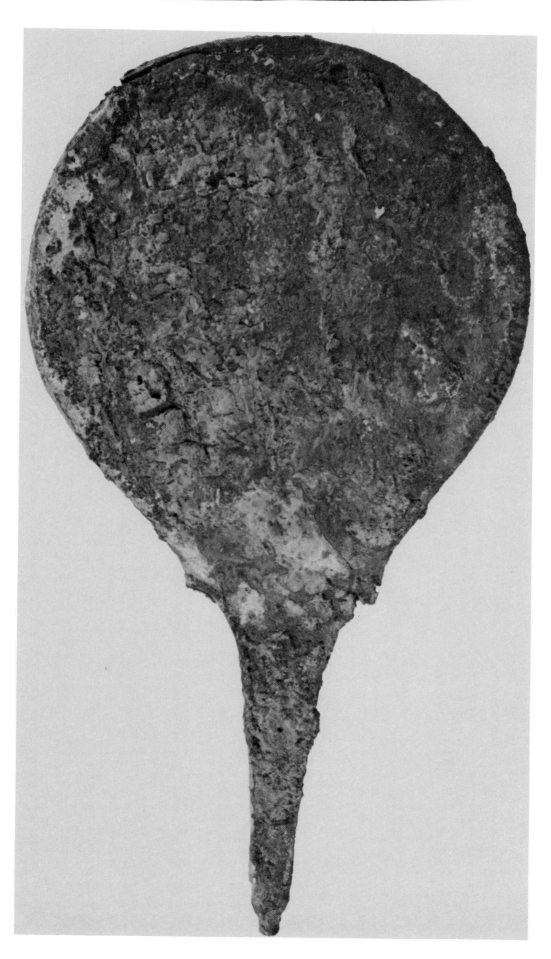

44b

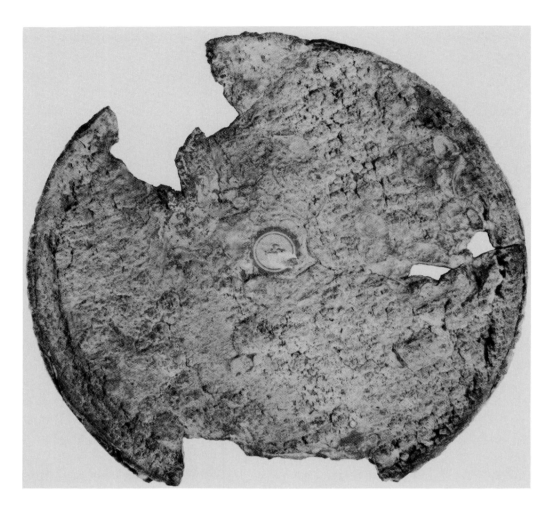

45a

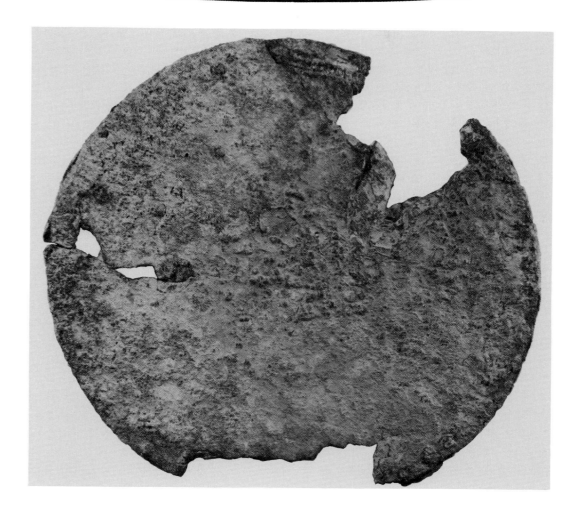

45b

PHOTOGRAPHIC CREDITS

APPENDIX

CHEMICAL ANALYSIS RESULTS

It was possible to analyze twenty-seven of the forty-four bronzes presented in this fascicle. Those not analyzed could not be sampled for a variety of reasons. Some were too thin or fragile; others were too corroded to provide a sample of clean bronze. The samples were normally taken from the tang or, in the case of handle mirrors, from the area just below the extension. Samples were obtained following the procedure described by M. M. HUGHES, M. R. COWELL, and P. T. CRADDOCK, *Atomic Absorption Techniques in Archaeology* in *Archaeometry* 18 (1976) 19–38.

Procedures: A known weight (5–15 mg ± 0.02 mg) of each bronze sample was digested in 2 mL aqua regia (1 volume nitric acid:3 volumes hydrochloric acid) by heating at 60°C. The prepared samples were diluted to 50 mL in volumetric flasks, and further dilutions were made as needed. Copper, tin, iron, cobalt, antimony, manganese, and bismuth were measured in the samples by using a technique of Inductively Coupled Plasma Emission Spectroscopy (ICP). This procedure is reported in G. F. WALLACE and P. BARRETT, *Analytical Methods Development for ICP Spectrometry* (Perkin-Elmer Corp., Norwalk, 1981). ICP operating conditions used were as follows:

Incident power	1250 watts
Reflected power	<5 watts
Plasma gas flow rate	14 liters/minute
Auxiliary gas flow rate	none
Nebulizer gas pressure	30 psi
Spectrometric viewing height	15 mm above load coil

Lead, nickel, and zinc were analyzed by flame atomic absorption spectrometry (see *Analytical Methods for Atomic Absorption Spectrophotometry* [Perkin-Elmer Corp., Norwalk, revised 1982]). Arsenic was measured by flameless atomic absorption spectrometry.

In some samples (Nos. **4, 15, 27, 37, 40**) the total recovery is somewhat more than 100 percent. In a few others (Nos. **1, 7, 8, 28, 41**) the total recovery is somewhat less than 100 percent. Possible explanations for these divergent recoveries are (1) contamination of the sample during collection, especially the intrusion of some exterior corrosion with interior core material; (2) insufficient sample size, which could cause experimental error. For those items showing low recovery, sample sizes ranged from 2.88 to 11.88 mg. Optimum sample size is 10 to 20 mg.

The results of these analyses are presented in Table 1.

In addition, twenty-three samples were analyzed by Electron Microprobe X-Ray Analysis. Some of these results appear in R. DE PUMA, *Engraved Etruscan Mirrors: Problems of Authenticity* in *Atti del Secondo Congresso Internazionale Etrusco* (Florence, 1986); others will be published elsewhere.

TABLE 1. Composition of bronze mirrors, percentage by weight

Mirror no.	Cu	Sn	Pb	As	Ni	Fe	Co	Zn	Ag	Sb	Mn	Bi
1	80.21	13.5	0.52	0.43	0.02	0.01	0.08	<0.02	0.02	0.14	<0.01	<0.01
3	83.43	15.94	1.17	0.13	0.06	0.03	<0.01	<0.01	0.07	0.35	<0.01	<0.01
4	88.93	12.71	0.11	0.14	<0.01	0.09	<0.01	<0.01	0.02	0.17	<0.01	<0.01
5	83.06	14.6	<0.10	0.22	0.06	0.01	0.05	<0.01	<0.01	0.10	<0.01	0.04
6	87.12	10.9	0.05	0.10	0.01	0.03	0.02	<0.01	0.02	0.11	<0.01	0.04
7	88.61	7.8	0.09	0.13	0.04	0.08	0.02	<0.01	0.03	0.10	<0.01	<0.01
8	77.83	14.5	0.37	0.43	0.16	0.50	0.09	<0.01	0.04	0.11	<0.01	<0.01
9	87.88	12.2	<0.14	0.05	<0.02	<0.02	0.03	<0.02	0.05	0.15	<0.01	<0.01
10	83.30	13.6	<0.17	0.48	0.05	0.10	0.05	<0.02	0.03	0.11	<0.01	0.04
13	88.27	10.8	0.04	0.22	0.04	0.11	0.06	<0.01	<0.01	0.11	<0.01	0.01
14	89.66	10.4	0.08	0.18	0.03	0.14	0.06	<0.01	0.02	0.12	<0.01	<0.01
15	89.53	11.6	0.02	0.05	0.03	0.05	0.03	<0.01	0.03	0.11	<0.01	<0.01
17	87.75	11.8	0.10	0.07	0.12	0.05	0.09	<0.01	0.03	0.10	<0.01	0.01
20	90.92	8.1	0.04	0.26	0.01	0.07	0.04	<0.01	0.03	0.11	<0.01	0.03
21	88.22	11.7	0.26	0.08	0.02	0.04	0.05	<0.01	0.05	0.11	<0.01	0.03
22	83.89	14.0	0.23	0.14	0.13	0.04	0.05	0.02	0.09	0.26	<0.01	0.04
23	85.09	10.0	3.47	0.16	0.03	0.08	0.06	<0.01	0.07	0.12	<0.01	0.07
26	91.04	8.0	1.19	0.16	0.05	0.03	0.03	<0.01	0.05	0.15	<0.01	0.04
27	85.91	14.6	0.04	0.39	0.03	0.11	0.10	<0.01	0.03	0.13	<0.01	0.02
28	80.86	13.8	0.17	0.10	0.04	0.16	0.07	0.04	0.05	0.12	<0.01	0.03
35	88.23	11.6	0.06	0.13	0.02	0.16	0.05	<0.01	0.03	0.11	<0.01	0.02
36	86.11	11.7	0.96	0.46	0.06	0.06	0.06	0.10	0.04	0.12	<0.01	0.04
37	88.91	12.7	0.08	0.33	0.06	0.02	0.10	<0.01	0.04	0.15	<0.01	0.01
38	87.33	11.7	0.72	0.21	0.03	0.41	0.13	0.07	0.07	0.13	<0.01	0.01
39	86.76	13.6	0.05	0.03	0.04	0.05	0.04	<0.01	0.06	0.13	<0.01	<0.01
40	89.63	11.03	<0.10	0.07	<0.01	0.24	<0.01	<0.01	0.01	<0.01	<0.01	<0.01
41	82.37	11.8	0.90	0.05	0.09	0.74	0.03	0.07	0.07	0.10	<0.01	<0.01

INDEXES

WITH REFERENCE TO CATALOGUE NUMBERS

EPIGRAPHICAL INDEX

CONCORDANCE with Gerhard, *ES*

CONCORDANCE OF CATALOGUE NUMBERS WITH RELATED PAGES AND FIGURES

Catalogue number	Figures	Page of cat. no.	Page of figures
Ann Arbor, Kelsey Museum			
1	1a–d	15–16	64–67
2	2a–d	16	68–71
Bloomington, Indiana University			
3	3a–d	17–18	72–75
4	4a–e	18–20	76–80
Chicago, Field Museum			
5	5a–d	21–22	82–85
6	6a–d	22	86–89
Chicago, Oriental Institute			
7	7a–d	23	90–93
8	8a–d	23–24	94–97
9	9a–d	24–25	98–101
10	10a–d	25	102–103
11	11a–b	25	104–105
12	12a–d	26	106–107
Cleveland Museum of Art			
13	13a–d	27	108–111
14	14a–e	28–29	112–116
15	15a–f	29–30	118–123
Columbia, University of Missouri			
16	16a–k	31–32	124–129
17	17a–d	32	130–133
18	18a–d	33	134–137
Crawfordsville, Wabash College			
19	19a–e	34–35	138–142
Dayton Art Institute			
20	20a–d	36–37	144–147
Detroit Institute of Arts			
21	21a–d	38–39	148–151
Iowa City, University of Iowa			
22	22a–d	40	152–155
Kansas City, Nelson-Atkins Museum			
23	23a–d	41–42	156–159

Catalogue number	Figures	Page of cat. no.	Page of figures
Lawrence, University of Kansas			
24	24a–d	43	160–163
Milwaukee Public Museum			
25	25a–d	44	164–167
Minneapolis, Institute of Arts			
26	26a–d	45–46	168–171
27	27a–d	46	172–175
Oberlin, Allen Memorial Art Museum			
28	28a–d	47–48	176–179
Omaha, Joslyn Art Museum			
29	29a	49	180
30	30a	49	181
31	31a–b	49	183
Rockford, Rockford College Art Collection			
32	32a–b	50	184–185
33	33a–d	50–51	186–189
34	34a–d	51	190–193
St. Louis Art Museum			
35	35a–d	52–53	194–197
36	36a–d	53–54	198–201
37	37a–d	54–55	202–205
Toledo Museum of Art			
38	38a–b	56	206–207
39	39a–d	56–58	208–211
ADDENDA:			
Bloomington, Indiana University			
40	40a–b	59	212–213
Chicago, Art Institute			
41	41a–e	60	214–218
Cincinnati Art Museum			
42	42a–c	61	220–222
43	43a–b	61	224–225
44	44a–b	61–62	226–227
45	45a–b	62	228–229